THE
HEALING
CUISINE
of CHINA

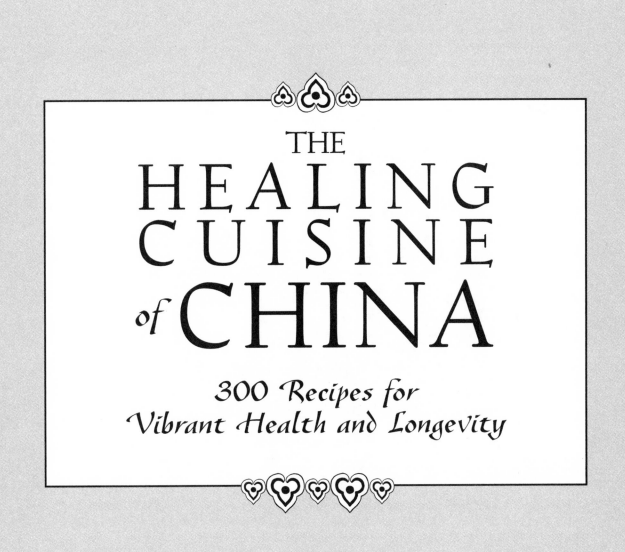

THE
HEALING
CUISINE
of CHINA

300 Recipes for
Vibrant Health and Longevity

ZHUO ZHAO & GEORGE ELLIS

Healing Arts Press
Rochester, Vermont

Healing Arts Press
One Park Street
Rochester, Vermont 05767
www.InnerTraditions.com
Healing Arts Press is a division of Inner Traditions International

Note to the reader: *This book is intended as an informational guide. The remedies, approaches, and
techniques described herein are meant to supplement, and not to be a substitute for, professional
medical care or treatment. They should not be used to treat a serious ailment
without prior consultation with a qualified health care professional.*

LIBRARY OF CONGRESS CATALOGING-IN-PUBLICATION DATA
Zhao, Zhuo, 1963–
The healing cuisine of China : 300 recipes for vibrant health and
longevity / Zhuo Zhao and George Ellis.
p. cm.
Includes index.
ISBN 0-89281-778-X (alk. paper)
1. Diet therapy—Recipes. 2. Cookery, Chinese. 3. Medicine, Chinese.
I. Ellis, George, 1949– . II. Title.
RM219.Z 1998
615.8′54′0951—dc21 98-42723
CIP

Printed and bound in Canada

10 9 8 7 6 5 4 3 2 1

Text design by Charlotte Tyler
Text layout by Virginia L. Scott
This book was typeset in Weiss and Cochin with Belwe as the display typeface

The questionnaire on pages 29–32 was adapted with permission of Sterling Publishing Co., Inc.,
387 Park Ave. South, New York, N.Y. 10016 from *Chinese System of Food Cures* by
Henry C. Lu, © 1986 by Henry C. Lu.

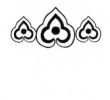

Contents

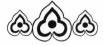

PREFACE

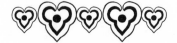

In China we take many facts about food, eating, and health habits for granted. When I first traveled to the United States in 1988, I was intrigued by many of the differences between Chinese and Western culture. Above all I was surprised by the differences in eating habits.

People in America seem to be obsessed with the concept of a healthy diet. Nutrition facts are printed on every jar, can, and package; everything is "fat free" or "low in cholesterol." People seem to know so much about food. They talk about organically grown foods, about fiber and vitamins and health. All this set me thinking about my own Chinese traditions.

When I lived in China I paid very little attention to tradition. Like most young people of my generation, I believed that everything Western was superior and that our Chinese culture was too old-fashioned to take seriously. Nevertheless, without realizing it I was absorbing many of my cultural traditions. In America, therefore, when I heard people rhapsodizing about low-fat vegetarian and "New Age" diets, I was perplexed. The precious organically grown tomatoes or cucumbers and the cooking methods that people so enthused about appeared to me to be perfectly ordinary. I soon realized that what was considered a normal diet in America must be something quite different from what I was used to.

Indeed, even "Chinese food" in America turned out to be different from what I expected. While there are thousands of Chinese restaurants in the United States, few of them serve the sort of food we expect to eat in China. In China we combine colors and flavors in ways that please the eyes and the palate. We balance our diet to consume a little of everything in the right combination and sequence: too much meat increases internal fire; too many raw vegetables give you a stomachache.

In China we always consider the health merits of what we eat. We don't like to deep-fry because frying is poison. We eat garlic because garlic cleanses the intestines, destroying harmful microorganisms. We select our foods according to the climate and time of year: when it is very hot, we eat cooling foods; in winter we eat warming foods.

We consume our drinks warm—even water is drunk hot. Hot water dissolves fats, assists digestion, and cures colds. As everybody in China knows, iced water blocks digestion. We drink soup at the end of our meals in order to clean the esophagus. Soup for us is a nutritious preparation in clear broth, nothing heavy or creamy. (Cream, milk, and cheeses have no place in Chinese cuisine.)

We know that you get a stomachache if you eat outdoors facing the wind, that green tea is important for burning fats, and that ginger kills germs.

Confucius said, "Ordinary people regard food as heaven." Eating is something that we do every day. The way we eat affects the way we live. Good, healthy cuisine not only improves the quality of our eating; it leads to a healthy body and mind, to harmony, and to a long life. When I stayed several months in America in 1993 I found myself thinking about food and the eating habits of our two cultures more than I had ever before. I decided then that I should write something about health and cuisine.

In my experience writing projects begin with a seed of an idea that makes its way onto a sheet of paper. From there it can either fizzle into oblivion or develop into a research project that engages most of one's waking life. The latter is what happened in this venture; the desire to write about Chinese ideas of health and cuisine led to two years of travel and research in China.

During the course of my research I realized that we Chinese have perhaps the vastest pharmacopoeia of food remedies of any country in the world. Other cultures hand down a few practical remedies from generation to generation. In China we have made a veritable science out of our traditional knowledge. In fact, we cannot separate traditional food remedies from traditional medicine in any meaningful way, beyond stating that the latter sometimes uses herbs and minerals that are harder to come by than raw foods.

I began my research by focusing on the Taoist theories underlying Chinese traditional medicine. At the same time I started collecting remedies and recipes. Some I tried on myself; some I tried on others. Most have proved amazingly efficient. I suffered from premenstrual cramps until I discovered the old Chinese remedy of ginger and brown sugar. Now I drink this broth regularly before my period and have, as a consequence, never needed to concern myself with the problem since. Whenever I suffer from a cough I drink daikon, ginger, and scallion soup to give relief. To anyone suffering from constipation I recommend honey, or, in more stubborn cases, fig tea. They work. When traveling rough in Tibet my husband and I protected ourselves by eating a clove of raw garlic with every meal. It may not be a coincidence that while everyone with us fell victim to the "runs," neither of us had the slightest problem.

Convinced by the evidence, we set about systematically recording and categorizing our facts. This led to a winter spent with a portable computer on a beach in India and then, with the help of my husband, George Ellis, to a manuscript. This book is the end result.

Zhuo Zhao
Arcata, California

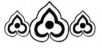

INTRODUCTION

To the Chinese, longevity is the greatest blessing of a good life. Consequently, it is a Chinese belief that the central duty of every man and woman is to cultivate health and fitness throughout one's entire lifetime. Out of that belief has developed a vast system of preventive methods for maintaining health, consisting of exercise, diet, rest, healthy living habits, and pre-emptive diagnoses.

When, despite efforts at prevention, disease does arise, the cause is sought in some underlying imbalance between the individual and his environment, and is corrected by proper eating. Only when all else fails does one resort to doctors and medicines.

This book is about the role of Chinese cuisine in the prevention and cure of disease. It also examines traditional Chinese methods of prevention through exercise and healthy living. It describes simple recipes, or "prescriptions" if you like, that anyone can prepare at home, with little expense, in order to cure many common and chronic ailments. Most of the ingredients we mention can be found in the nearest supermarket; a few may have to be obtained from a store specializing in Oriental foods.[1] None of the remedies in this book require particular attention to dosages or mode of preparation: all the ingredients but one are categorized by the Chinese as "high-grade" drugs. Basically, this classification means that they are food items: wholesome beyond their purely medicinal function, they can therefore be taken continuously over a period of time with no ill effects.[2] Examples of such ingredients are garlic, ginger, celery, and coriander, or, when we get more complicated, jujube (Chinese dates) or cardamom seeds.

Traditionally the line separating "food" from "medicine" has never been clear. In

1

the same way there has never been a precise division between popular home remedies and official Chinese medicine. People in China take whatever is available locally to cure their ailments. Even today, more than 80 percent of the population in China live off the land. They eat what they grow in their own fields and when they fall ill they take the traditional remedies of the land. The people have been there for millennia; experience has taught them or their forefathers, or their forefathers' forefathers. Sometimes by pure chance, or on the basis of an intuitive hunch, someone might stumble across a new and unexpected therapeutic effect of a common spice, fruit, or herb. They tell their friends and family. Others try it. Word spreads until the new remedy comes to the notice of one of China's traditional wandering doctors. He tries it himself, uses it on his patients, and records it for posterity.[3] In this way a home remedy becomes an official remedy. This process of testing and transition is called the *empirical method*. Over a single lifetime the empirical method does not go far. Over nearly five thousand years of recorded history, the trials and errors of a people bent on staying physically fit must surely yield results.

These results form the basis of the rules, prescriptions, and remedies in this book, which we have collected from original Chinese sources, ancient and modern, published and unpublished. We hope that by publishing them in English we may both further the understanding of Chinese medical theory and practice in the English-speaking world and, above all, provide access to centuries of clinical experience that may improve the quality of life for anybody willing to try the ancient Chinese way to health through food.

There are several circumstances in which this book might prove useful. You may wish simply to prepare good, wholesome Chinese cuisine with a view to keeping you and your family healthy. Or you may wish to follow a Chinese dietary and fitness regimen for generic disease prevention or for weight control. The suggested recipes and prescriptions will provide relief from many minor and chronic health problems—a headache, a blocked nose, an allergy—that often do not merit the time and expense of a visit to the doctor. Other conditions might require surgery (a hemorrhoid problem, for instance) but your preference would be to try alternatives first. There are occasions when you might be dealing with a common illness—influenza or a cold—when you may not wish to poison your body with chemical medicines, the ill effects of which might take at least two weeks to wear off. Or you might be suffering from one of those ailments, terminal or insignificant, most of them chronic, that Western allopathic medicine simply cannot cure. Chinese medicine cannot guarantee results either, but some of these conditions have been known to regress, if not to disappear, under the influence of Chinese natural remedies. Hypertension, asthma, obesity, anorexia, psoriasis, multiple sclerosis, and some forms of cancer are but a few of these.

At a time when dissatisfaction in the United States with mainstream allopathic medicine seems to be on the rise and when leading research institutes, as well as many of the "alternative" therapies, seem to do little more than contradict everything we knew last year—Is cholesterol bad or isn't it? Are eggs good for the liver? Does alcohol damage the heart or guard against coronary disease?—it seems only reasonable to pay attention to what one-fifth of humanity has been preaching, and practicing, for millennia.

This is not to say that one should go

completely in the other direction and put wide-eyed trust exclusively in Chinese medicine. It has its limits. First and foremost, Chinese natural medicine takes time to act, often taxing the patience of all but its most resolute adherents. Secondly, it fails to deliver on some occasions when a mere two-week course of antibiotics could provide a quick and permanent cure.[4] Finally, there is the problem of understanding the theoretical basis of traditional Chinese medicine. When discussing the effects of foods and recipes we refer to imbalances of Yin and Yang or the Five Elements, to "hot" and "cold" syndromes, to the "evil wind," and to "upward," "downward," "outward," and "inward" movements of foods and drugs. Furthermore, Chinese medicine seems to ignore some of the basics that Westerners take for granted. It makes no mention of familiar terms like *bacteria, viruses, vitamins,* or *enzymes.* This can be confusing.

In order to render the concepts of traditional Chinese medicine meaningful we have attempted, in chapter 1, to illustrate as synthetically as possible the underlying theories behind traditional Chinese beliefs regarding health and illness.

Chapter 2 examines the exogenous and endogenous pathogenic causes of disease,

and also discusses some of the doubts and misconceptions that might arise from attempting to fit Chinese theory into the Western paradigm. Both the successes and failures of Chinese medicine are considered.

The rest of the book is about Chinese food remedies themselves. Chapter 3 describes the methods of preparing and eating traditional Chinese cuisine for health. It also provides the reader with a questionnaire for recognizing his or her physical characteristics, with a view to selecting the most suitable balanced diet for perfect health.

Chapter 4 looks at the ingredients used in the recipes and prescriptions. Chapter 5 provides the reader with recipes and prescriptions for curing common ailments. Chapter 6 takes the form of a cookbook as it instructs the reader in the ancient art of preparing easy but complete meals for health and longevity.

Finally, chapter 7 describes traditional Chinese *qi gong* exercises as a means of keeping healthy.

It is with the traditional Chinese augury of a long and healthy life that we leave you to the exploration of the joys and proven health benefits of Chinese therapeutic cuisine. *Chang ming bai sui*—A long life of one hundred years!

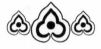

Chapter 1

THE ORIGINS AND THEORY OF CHINESE MEDICAL KNOWLEDGE

According to legend, sometime between 2697 and 2597 B.C. the renowned first Yellow Emperor, Huangdi, otherwise known as Shen-nong or "King of farming," tasted one hundred wild herbs and grasses.[1] He was trying to ascertain their values as cures to various ailments from which he was presumably suffering. As a consequence, the Yellow Emperor is credited as being the first person in China to institute the art of healing.

For the following two thousand years people continued to test herbs, fruits, fungi, and barks on themselves, as well as on some unfortunate patients, and to record the results. Gradually this hit-or-miss approach—tempered, we would hope, by the observation of animals' eating habits and by some sort of primitive ideas about physiology and illness—led to the development of a comprehensive theory of health, disease, and treatment.[2] Inevitably, medical theory was made to fit into contemporary beliefs about the nature of the world. These beliefs have come down to us

under the name Taoism—pronounced **dow**-izm—meaning "the Way."

By the so-called Warring States period (475–221 B.C.), Taoist medical theory was sufficiently developed to warrant the systematic compilation of all the then-known facts about human anatomy and physiology, and disease pathology, prevention, diagnosis, and treatment. The compilers of the first such record appear to have been various medics working as a group. Either because they were following the fashion of the times (attributing everything to ancient origins), playing modest, or seeking some sort of legitimacy for wild new theories, the authors called their book Huangdi's (the Yellow Emperor's) Internal Classic (*Huangdi Nei Jing*). They wrote it as if it were a dialogue between the Yellow Emperor and his chief counselor, Qi Bo. Whatever the origin and true antiquity of the ideas presented by them, the authors of Huangdi's Internal Classic laid the foundation for Chinese medical theory and practice a foundation that is valid to this day.

The *Huangdi Nei Jing* is divided into two parts. The first part, Su Wen (Plain Questions), considers human anatomy, physiology, and pathology within the Taoist theory of *yin* and *yang* and the Five Elements. The remedies it espouses are principally herbal. It is on the basis of the Plain Questions that all subsequent medical theory was founded.

The second part is called Ling Shu, or Miraculous Pivot. It discusses the anatomical theory of vital energy (*qi*) channels within the body and regulation of the circulating qi and the Five Elements by means of acupuncture.

THE TAOIST THEORY OF YIN AND YANG

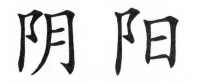

Figure 1: Energy of the moon and energy of the sun, signifying Yin and Yang

Taoism is a theory of the equilibrium of all nature. Based on early animism and formalized in approximately 500 B.C. by the writings of Lao Tzu (Old Sage), and subsequently by those of Zhuang Zi (Chuang-Tzu), Taoism envisages a world in which the ideal condition is harmony—a perfect balance between human beings and the environment, and among human beings themselves.[3] Taoism emphasizes relationships between opposites, aiming toward the perfection of equilibrium. The equilibrium itself is never permanent. Life is an ongoing process of give and take, of energy

absorption and energy loss. As a consequence, every living process in nature is characterized by conflict, accommodation, and complementarity. Today we call this *homeostasis*.

The fundamental forces of the Taoist world are named Yin and Yang. Yin means "in the shade;" Yang translates as "in the sunlight." Extrapolating from this basic concept Yin and Yang came to mean, repectively, darkness and light, moon and sun, passivity and activity, female and male, cold and heat, inside and outside, down and up, left and right, negative and positive, substance and function, emptiness and fullness, hidden and exposed.

Just as the natural world is characterized by the antagonism and flow of Yin and Yang, so is the human body. Indeed, Taoism would find no reason to differentiate between the natural world and that of human experience. To the Taoist, dualism was the greatest error. Instead, Taoist philosophy suggests that we are an integral part of the whole, a flux and flow of vital energy within a larger energy. Today we would call this *holism*.

Thus, when the authors of Huangdi's Internal Classic set out to study human physiology, they based their concept of health on the equilibrium of Yin and Yang. In chapter 5 of the Su Wen (Plain Questions) they wrote: "Yin and Yang are the law of Heaven and Earth, the outline of everything, the parents of change, the origin of birth and destruction."

The active and dynamic processes of the human body—such as eating, digesting, and metabolizing—they called Yang. The passive functions—such as breathing and blood circulation—are seen as Yin. Diseases were also differentiated between Yin and Yang. Diseases that affect the bodily functions, are virulent in nature, and progress rapidly within the body or ascend from the viscera to the head are considered to be Yang. Those that are organic, lie dormant, are degenerative, are characterized by low activity, or descend from the upper part of the body are Yin. The herbs taken to cure these diseases are, in their turn, also differentiated between Yin and Yang.

Yin and Yang in human health, as in all of nature, are both interdependent and mutually restricting. They rely on each other for their own being. Each contains within it the seed of the other. Where one increases the other decreases; when one reaches its peak the other emerges. These

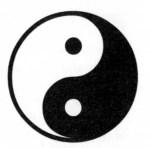

Figure 2: The symbol of Yang and Yin. The upper function, Yang, is in the light and is therefore white. The lower function, Yin, represents the shade and darkness. Yet, as symbolized by the dots within each form, Yang and Yin each contains within itself the seed of its opposite; each is born from the other. When one increases the other decreases.

concepts are expressed in pictorial form by the well-known symbol of Yin and Yang's circular complementarity.

The Yin and Yang aspects within a living body are in constant interaction, and one always increases at the expense of the other. Activity is Yang; nutrient substances are, in general, Yin. Thus any activity—running, walking, talking—that consumes energy from digested nutrients lessens Yin and, as a result, increases Yang. On the other hand, the metabolism of those same nutrient substances (Yin) depletes the functional energy (Yang) and consequently increases Yin at the expense of Yang. In ordinary circumstances the mutual depletion and increase of Yin and Yang balances itself out. Unusual circumstances—too much activity, too much food, impaired metabolism, or too little activity or food—create an imbalance. In the long term, the imbalance can lead to disease.

Yet Yin and Yang do not exert their influence purely as vital functions. They are, according to Chinese medical theory, attributes of parts of the body as well. Yang is above and Yin is below, therefore the top half of the human body is considered to be Yang and everything below the waist is Yin. Yang is outward and Yin inward. The inside of our body is Yin and the outside Yang. Similarly, the back is Yang and the front Yin, the sides are Yang and the central portion is Yin.

What is true of the body as a whole is also considered valid for the vital organs. In Chinese traditional theory the vital organs are divided, according to their functions, into *zang* (generating and storing organs) and *fu* (transforming, transporting, and distributing organs). Generating and storing is considered a Yin activity, therefore the five zang organs (*wu zang*)—the heart, the liver, the spleen, the lungs, and the kidneys—are all considered Yin. Transforming, transporting, and distributing are said to be Yang activities. It follows, therefore, that the six fu organs (*liu fu*)—the gall bladder, the stomach, the small intestine, the large intestine, the urinary bladder, and the three main body cavities (*san jiao*)—are considered Yang.

Because Yin and Yang are everywhere

complementary and interdependent, the parts of the human body that are Yang also contain aspects of Yin within themselves, and vice versa. What this means is that within the heart there exists a Yang function too: pumping blood through the body. Yet even within that Yang function of pumping lies a passive Yin function: blood circulation. Within that Yin of circulation can be found the Yang of nutrition to the vital organs. The organs themselves are Yin, which takes us back to where we started from: the heart.

The point is that Yang and Yin are interdependent and complementary to one another. They cannot exist in isolation. Each contains the seed and essence of the other. Within Yang there is Yin, within that Yin another Yang, and so on and so on to infinity.

As the Plain Questions of Huangdi's Internal Classic puts it: "In any one function, Yin and Yang could amount to ten in number, be extended to one hundred, to one thousand, to ten thousand and even to the infinite."

All healthy activities of the human body arise from the maintenance of this dynamic equilibrium between Yin and Yang. For example, when the lungs expand and contract they are performing a Yang function, as *all* activity is Yang. The activity of breathing is based on the substance of the lungs—substance is Yin. Therefore the Yang and the Yin of breathing are interdependent. When one is healthy, the other flourishes; when either one diminishes—through inactivity (improper breathing), malnutrition, or some external factor such as injury or viral disease—the other aspect withers.

The Plain Questions section of Huangdi's Internal Classic states: "When Yin keeps balance with Yang and both

maintain a normal condition of qi (vital energy), then health will be high-spirited. A separation of Yin and Yang will lead to the exhaustion of essential qi."

The causes of imbalance between Yin and Yang are many and varied. Traditional Chinese medical theory regards external pathogens (xie qi, literally, "incorrect" or "evil energy") and the state of the body's resistance to these external pathogens as the major causes of imbalance. Xie qi (pathogens) are seen as external factors. They can arise from climatic aberrations, lack of adaptation to a changed environment, or from the "six excesses." These excesses are wind (frequently referred to as "evil wind"), cold, heat, firelike heat, dampness, and dryness. Pathogens can also be either Yin or Yang in nature. A Yang pathogen—too much dry heat for example—will decrease the body's Yang functions. Because of their interdependence, impairment of a Yang function weakens the generation and development of Yin as well. A so-called heat syndrome results. A Yin pathogen on the other hand will diminish Yin, leading to damage of bodily Yang with a resulting cold syndrome. (As a general rule, Yin excess causes a cold syndrome and Yang excess gives rise to a heat syndrome.)

Therapy will be based on correcting the Yin/Yang imbalance. If excess Yang is the cause of a heat syndrome, it is necessary to nourish the weakened Yin by ingesting cooling Yin foods and herbs. Conversely, when a cold syndrome damages the body's Yang, Yin becomes preponderant and recourse must be made to hot, Yang foods and medicines. The general principle is thus: Treat Yang diseases with Yin foods and treat Yin disorders with Yang foods.

In order to appreciate the complexities of traditional Chinese food therapy, however, more understanding is called for. In addition to grasping the concept of Yin and Yang imbalances, we need to know something about the Five Elements of nature and their relationships to the five zang and the six fu organs, the concept of qi, and the three causes of disease before delving into the principles of using food and herbal medicines.

五行　THE FIVE ELEMENTS

As we have said, according to Taoism everything in nature is either Yin or Yang. Everything in nature is also seen as being constituted by a combination of the five basic elements. This is similar to medieval European and Indian concepts of the five humors (earth, air, water, fire, and ether), though the elements themselves are different. The five Chinese elements, the *wu xing*, are Metal (Jin), Wood (Mu), Water (Shui), Fire (Huo), and Earth (Tu).

Just as the mutual restriction and enhancement of Yin and Yang is important to understanding Chinese concepts of health, disease, and corrective therapy, appreciating the complex interdependence between the Five Elements is necessary in order to interpret the relationship between human physiology and pathology and the natural environment. For, despite the name, the concepts behind the Five Elements are more complex than the purely material ones of medieval alchemy.

The elements may be referred to simply as metal, wood, water, fire, and earth, but, in actual fact, they are not seen as mere objects. They are more appropriately regarded as attributes and functions. The Chinese term for them, *wu xing*, does not mean "elements" at all. *Wu* means "five" and

xing can be translated as "movement" or "that which causes action." "Metal" therefore represents the properties of strength and firmness, of cleansing and destroying. "Wood" is a shorthand way of expressing the functions of germination, extension, softness, and harmony. "Water" represents cold, dampness, and flowing downward. "Fire" signifies heat and flaring. "Earth" refers to the processes of growing, nourishing, and changing.[4]

These processes are continuously enhancing, restricting, and subjugating one another in much the same way as Yin and Yang complement and limit one another in all natural phenomena. The relationship between the Elements is a precise one; it exists wherever the Elements themselves induce activity. It exists, therefore, in the changing seasons, in the ebb and flow of climate, in life itself. It also exists within the functions of the human body.

Our internal organs, our organs of sense, our tissues, even our emotional life, all are characterized by specific Elements/functions. The functions of the heart, for example, are regarded as belonging to the element Fire. Fire is heat and energy, and the heart is regarded as the organ that imparts energy to all the others. Without the Fire-heart, the human body cannot survive. Fire is nourished by Wood; the heart, therefore, is nourished by the principal organ of the Wood element, the liver. As a consequence, the health of the liver is regarded as indispensable to the well-being of the heart. On the other hand, Fire is extinguished by Water. It follows that if the kidneys, whose element is Water, fail to function properly, the heart is affected.

These basic relationships between the Five Elements are described as "generating" and "subjugating." The order of generation between the Five Elements is this: Wood generates Fire, Fire generates Earth, Earth generates Metal, Metal generates Water, and Water generates Wood. This is frequently referred to as the *mother-child relationship*. In the control cycle, Water subjugates Fire, Fire subjugates Metal, Metal subjugates Wood, Wood subjugates Earth, and Earth subjugates Water. These basic generating and subjugating relationships are illustrated in figure 3.

At the level of the Five Elements, illness is characterized by a breakdown of the equilibrium between generation and subjugation. When one of the Elements becomes overactive it tends to break out of its normal generating/subjugating relationships. Strong Fire, for example, will violate Water, consuming it and turning it into steam instead of being quenched by it. At the same time it will subjugate Metal beyond its ordinary capacity, encroaching on it and threatening to destroy it. These pathological relationships are expressed as "violating" and "encroaching" or "subjugating" to the extreme. In disequilibrium situations, including human illness, Fire violates Water and destroys Metal; Water violates Earth and extinguishes Fire; Earth violates Wood and dries up Water; Wood violates Metal and consumes Earth; Metal violates Fire and utterly destroys Wood. These relationships are illustrated in figure 4.

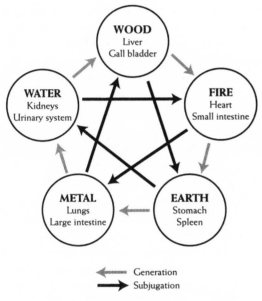

Figure 3: Healthy balance between the Elements and their corresponding organs

Through these mutually enhancing and restrictive relationships, a second level of equilibrium is achieved beyond that of Yin and Yang. According to the *Lei Jing*, a Ming dynasty commentary on *Huangdi Nei Jing*, "If there is no generation, there is no growth and development. If there is no restriction, then endless growth and development will become harmful."[5] This concept is central to the Chinese theory of good health.

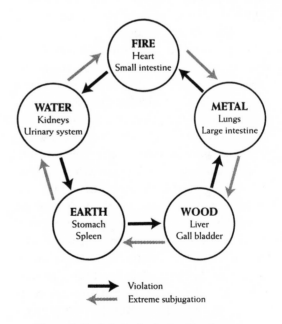

Figure 4: Pathological relationships between the Elements and their corresponding organs

When consulting with a new patient a Chinese physician will observe, ask about symptoms, and test the pulse in order to base his or her diagnosis on the relative forces of Yin and Yang as well as on these primary relationships of generation, subjugation, violation, and extreme subjugation between the Elements and the internal organs. The doctor will, however, also inquire into the patient's diet and consider the climate, locality, and time of year. No one exists in isolation from the environment; everything about us is charged with the properties of the Five Elements. Therefore the food we eat, the air we breathe, the climate—our entire surroundings—affect us in one way or another. Each of the seasons belongs to a different Element, as does each direction. (In Chinese philosophy there are five of both: spring, summer, late summer, autumn, and winter; north, south, east, west, and center.) It follows, therefore, that the careful doctor must consider all these factors when deciding on the severity of the symptoms and on the appropriate treatment.

What this boils down to, in effect, is that if you are unwell you must first try to understand the relationship between the diseased part of you, your emotions, the time of year, the part of the world you happen to be in, the climate, and what you've been eating. If, to take a light-hearted example, your lips erupt with cold sores in New Orleans in the summer where you've been singing at Preservation Hall and indulging your sweet tooth, you may be suffering from nothing more complicated than an excess of the Earth element. The Earth—or transforming—Element is abundant in the late summer, in damp climates, in song, and in sweet food. Its excess affects the stomach and the mouth. The remedy would be counteracting Earth with its subjugating element, Wood. In order to achieve that you might move to Boston.

More practically, you might eat a diet of greens and cool, sour food, and your troubles would likely disappear. The east, a windy climate, the color green, and sour food are all attributes of the Wood element.

This is, of course, a far-fetched example, but it serves to illustrate the point. The elements in the environment, those within you, and those in your food interact continuously to create situations that can lead either to better health or to debility and disease.

Tables 1 and 2 list characteristics of the various Elements within the human body and in nature. This information can help in diagnosing basic imbalances. The effects of imbalances between the Five Elements within the human body can give rise to many and varied symptoms. For example, a lack of qi (vital energy) in any one organ/function may set off a chain reaction whereby the organ/function normally generated by the weakened organ is depleted of energy and the organ it is supposed to subjugate increases its qi to the point that it stagnates. The outcome is usually malaise and then disease.

Let us look at each of the Five Elements and their five corresponding zang (generating and storing organs) to understand how this happens. (Throughout this discussion you may want to refer back to figure 3 illustrating the generation and subjugation cycles.)

木 Mu

"A single tree," (i.e., Wood)—to germinate
Corresponding zang organ: liver
Organ, tissues, and sense organ affected by
  Wood: The gall bladder, the tendons, the eyes

In China, to explain the function of Wood it is said that "Trees like to spread their branches freely." The liver therefore "germinates" vital energy (qi) and spreads it

TABLE 1: HUMAN PHYSIOLOGY RELATIVE TO THE FIVE ELEMENTS

Element:	Wood	Fire	Earth	Metal	Water
Attribute:	Germination	Growth	Transformation	Reaping	Storage
Bodily organs:	Liver	Heart	Spleen	Lung	Kidney
	Gall bladder	Small intestine	Stomach	Large intestine	Urinary system
Sense organ:	Eye	Tongue	Mouth	Nose	Ear
Tissue:	Tendons	Vessels	Muscles	Skin and hair	Bone
Emotion:	Anger	Joy	Worry	Melancholy/grief	Fear
Sound:	Shouts	Laughter	Singing	Crying	Mourning
Flavor:	Sour	Bitter	Sweet	Pungent	Salty

TABLE 2: NATURAL PHENOMENA RELATIVE TO THE FIVE ELEMENTS

Element:	Wood	Fire	Earth	Metal	Water
Color:	Green	Red	Yellow	White	Black
Climate:	Wind	Humid heat	Dampness	Dryness	Cold
Direction:	East	South	Center	West	North
Voice tones:*	Jiao	Zheng	Gong	Shang	Yu
Season:	Spring	Summer	Late summer	Autumn	Winter

* Traditionally the Chinese physician based his diagnosis in part on the timbre and tone of voice of the patient. The names of the tones are untranslatable—they correspond to our *do, re, mi, fa,* and *so. La* and *si (ti)* do not exist because the ancient Chinese system envisaged only five tones.

throughout the body. When Wood flourishes it generates Fire by transforming food into qi. The liver Fire feeds the heart, which is itself of the Fire element. The heart Fire then generates the Earth element, which corresponds to the spleen. The Earth element is subjugated by Wood; the liver, therefore, directly inhibits the function of the spleen, as well as contributing to it through heart Fire.

A weak Wood element leads to a feeble Fire element, resulting in headaches, dizziness, flushed features and, occasionally, mental imbalance. As a consequence, the spleen can become dysfunctional as well.

When the Wood element in the liver is too strong, it results in Fire of the liver. The Metal element is consequently subjugated to the extreme (see figure 3). Metal element resides in the lungs. The lungs are therefore impaired by Fire in the liver, leading to a dry cough and chest pains.

Foods that correct these imbalances

would do so by acting directly on the underlying weakness. A dysfunctional liver would be treated by nourishing the weak Wood element. Some Wood-nourishing foods are trout, cheese, and many fruits and berries, such as grapes, lychee, mango, olives, pears, plums, raspberries, strawberries, tangerines, and tomatoes. Sour flavors help Wood to germinate and grow; vinegar, therefore, is ideal for exerting a strengthening influence on Wood. Because of the correspondence between human and animal organs, fresh and healthy animal liver is also considered to be a good remedy for weakness in the liver. Celery, egg yolk, chicken, plums, and peppermint are also valid.

When the Wood element is excessively strong it leads to Fire in the liver and to a consequent stagnation of qi in this organ. The main treatment is to circulate the stagnant qi and to allow the liver to rest; alcohol and heavy and oily foods should therefore be avoided. Because Metal is subjugated to the extreme by Fire in the liver, Metal must be built up in order reestablish equilibrium. The foods that are most suitable for this are the herbs and spices: basil, bay leaf, black and white pepper, capers, cayenne, coriander, dill seed, garlic, ginger, marjoram, mustard greens, nutmeg, rosemary, and peppermint.

火 Huo

"A flame generated by the contact of two flint-stones," (i.e., Fire)—to grow
Corresponding zang organ: heart
Organ, tissues, and sense organ affected by Fire:
The small intestine, the blood vessels, the tongue

In traditional Chinese medicine the heart is the governing organ of the body. It is thought to be the seat of the self, of spirit and vitality. As such, the health of the entire mind-body system depends on the health of the heart.

The heart belongs to the Fire element. It is generated by Wood (the liver) and, in turn generates Earth (the spleen and the stomach). On the other hand it is suppressed by Water (the kidneys). When the heart Fire is depleted, through lack of qi from the liver for example, the result is poor digestion and diarrhea (the spleen and stomach depend on heart Fire for health) and low energy in the whole body. When the kidneys fail to function normally the heart is directly affected, resulting in insomnia and emotional problems.

When, on the other hand, the heart Fire burns with excessive heat, the "flames" are said to flare upward, resulting in flushed features, headache, sore throat, bleeding gums, abscesses in the mouth, and bloodshot eyes. Excessive fire also melts Metal (the lung), thus injuring this organ.

Foods that nourish Fire are tangerine, lettuce, papaya, pumpkin, scallion, and rye. Being the flavor associated with Fire, bitter foods also strengthen Fire. The organs that correspond to Fire are the heart and the small intestine; any food that strengthens these will, as a consequence, affect Fire. Some heart-nourishing foods are mung bean, egg yolk, ginseng, licorice, longans, persimmon, and red and cayenne pepper.

Excessive Fire (or inflammation) leads to indigestion, constipation, and the stagnation of blood. This condition may be tempered by strengthening Water, the element that subjugates Fire. Suitable foods to this end are water chestnut, banana, and tangerine peel. Drinking plenty of water is also useful.

土 Tu

"Two layers of soil from which a plant grows,"
  (i.e., Earth)—to transform
Corresponding zang organ: spleen
Organ, tissues, and sense organ affected by Earth:
  The stomach, the muscles, the mouth

Earth (the spleen) is generated by Fire and regulated by Wood (the liver). The function of the Earth element is to transform; the spleen is therefore involved in the digestion and assimilation of food and in the subsequent storing and distribution of nutrients. It generates Metal (the lungs) and subjugates Water (the kidneys).

The Earth element thrives in warm, dry environments and suffers in cold and damp ones. When the spleen is weak it fails to control normal water metabolism, resulting in urinary problems and, frequently, in diarrhea.

Sweet foods correspond to the Earth and therefore nourish this element. Since sweet is the most common flavor, Earth and spleen-nourishing foods are plentiful. They include most ripe fruits, nuts, and vegetables, as well as seafood, meats, tofu, beans, potatoes, rice, and, of course, honey and sugar. Sour foods are detrimental to a weakened Earth because they nourish Wood and can thus subjugate Earth. In terms of the corresponding organs, a dysfunction of the liver (Wood) will give rise to a pathological condition in the spleen and stomach (Earth).

If you suffer from urinary problems caused by weak Earth, you should eat plenty of sweet foods. All ripe fruits exert a positive effect, but watermelon is perhaps the ideal; besides nourishing Earth with its sweetness, its high water content serves to flush out toxins and clear the urinary passage.

金 Jin

"Two gold nuggets hidden in the earth,"
  (i.e., Metal)—to reap
Corresponding zang organ: lungs
Organ, tissues, and sense organ affected by Metal:
  The large intestine, the skin and hair, the nose

The lungs and the large intestine both correspond to the Metal element. The main function of the lungs is in respiration—absorbing qi, the vital energy of air, and circulating it throughout the body.

From the Five Elements point of view, Metal generates Water and subjugates Wood. The lungs, therefore, contribute to normal water metabolism and regulate the functions of the kidneys. When the lungs are diseased, the kidneys (Water) are directly affected. In China it is said that "a muffled gong does not sound," a reference to the fact that when Metal is attacked by external pathogens, the lungs suffer and hoarseness or low voice ensues.

Because of the correspondence between Metal, the lungs and large intestine, and the pungent flavor, any disease that weakens the lungs or intestines may be treated with pungent—Metal element—foods. These include pumpkin, leek, rosemary, fennel, and red and black pepper. However, since Metal is generated by Earth, eating sweet Earth foods will also nourish the lungs and large intestine: white mushrooms, grapes, and persimmon, for example, are sweet in flavor and generate fluids that lubricate the lungs. Other favored foods for treating the lungs are carrot and radish, basil, licorice, cinnamon twig, garlic, ginger, peppermint, scallion, mustard leaf, olive, peanut, walnut, water chestnut, and tangerine.

The large intestine is also favorably affected by consuming tofu and other soybean products, figs, spinach, lettuce, Chinese cabbage, freshwater fish, maize, cucumber, eggplant, nutmeg, and black and white pepper.

水 Shui

"Liquid flowing downward," (i.e., Water)—
  to store
Corresponding zang organ: kidneys
Organs, tissues, and sense organ affected by
  Water: The urinary system, the bones, the ear

The kidneys correspond to Water. Water tends to flow downward, thus exerting influence on the lower (Yin) half of the body. It is therefore believed that sexual debility in both sexes is directly attributable to weakness of the kidneys.

Water generates Wood and subjugates Fire. When Water fails to provide Wood with sufficient nourishment, the liver suffers. As we have seen the liver generates Fire, which maintains a healthy heart. Weak Water energy therefore affects both the distribution of vital energy throughout the body and the proper functioning of the heart. The resulting symptoms are pain in the lumbar region, digestive problems, wind, diarrhea, swelling of the feet and legs, irritability, and insomnia.

Drinking large quantities of water is not the solution, nor is the intake of a lot of salt, despite the fact that salty flavor corresponds to Water. To nourish the kidneys, seeds and nuts such as sesame, caraway, dill seed, fennel, star anise, soybean, walnut, chestnut, and lotus seed may be eaten. Other nourishing foods for the kidneys are freshwater fish, cuttlefish, eel, egg yolk, mutton, pork, and wheat products.

Because of its flowing nature, Water is particularly sensitive to imbalances in all the Elements and organs. If a weak Earth fails to control Water, normal Water metabolism is impaired, resulting in diarrhea and edema. Metal, too, must be strengthened so as to properly nourish Water. Bitter foods such as grapefruit, orange, and tangerine peel; bitter gourd; radish leaf; asparagus; and celery exert a positive effect.

❖ ❖ ❖

For our purposes, the point of this discussion is not to memorize or even pay too studious attention to the precise interactions between the various organs and Elements. It is to remember that whenever we resort to Chinese food or medical therapies, whether for maintaining health or for curing disease, we should consider the mutually regulating interrelationships that exist between all of the Five Elements and their corresponding organs. While this may seem daunting to those readers unschooled in traditional Chinese medicine, it will suffice to bear in mind the simple fact that often, in order to treat a symptom connected with one part of the body, we may have to act on an underlying weakness somewhere else. Or, to put it the way we do in China: You must treat the mother to cure the child.

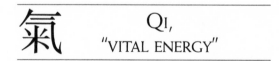

QI, "VITAL ENERGY"

Yin and Yang and the Five Elements are not material things. They are processes. As such they involve energy in all their functions and interactions. This energy the Taoists call qi, commonly translated as "vital energy" or "essential energy." Qi involves both function and substance.

Qi is the energy that supports life. It comes into being with life itself and is replenished through food and the inspiration of air. Congenital qi, *yuan qi*, arouses and promotes the activity of the Five Elements and the organs of the body. Qi from air and food descends through the energy channels of the body to be stored in the center of the body, the *dan tian*, about four inches below the navel. From the dan tian qi circulates both in the blood and in the conduit channels and collaterals (the meridians of acupuncture theory). Wherever qi goes it nourishes the organs of the body with its life-giving force.

Strong, unobstructed flow of qi ensures life and health; weak qi is generally the precursor of illness. Any organ or part of the body to which the flow of qi is obstructed will weaken, leading to the organ's withering. As a result, qi stagnates elsewhere in the body and Yin and Yang and the Five Elements become imbalanced. Disease is the inevitable outcome.

Too little or stagnant qi manifests in various ways according to the part of the body being affected. Shallow breathing, for example, indicates lack of qi in the lungs; poor appetite and impaired digestion mean that stomach qi is weak. Hence the importance of maintaining healthy, flowing qi. This is accomplished through diet and through qi gong, or qi control exercises, which we discuss later in the book.

Although unrecognized by allopathy, qi is fundamental to Chinese medical theory. It is the vital force that sustains life and guarantees good health by oxygenating the blood and nourishing the organs and the lymphatic and nervous systems. Without the concept of qi Chinese medicine would be at a loss to explain the workings of acupuncture, the positive effects of the qi gong system of exercises, the benefits of massage and acupressure, even the fundamental questions relating to the nature of health and of life itself.

Qi, therefore, is referred to continuously both in Chinese medical treatises and in popular discussions about life, health, and disease; we too shall consider the qi-nourishing properties of food throughout this book.

Whether you wish to accept the Chinese belief that qi is something substantial, or instead prefer to interpret it in terms of oxygen and the processes of oxygenation or as another way of talking about energy, it is important to understand that, from the Chinese point of view, nourishing qi, the health of qi, and qi circulation are as important—and perhaps more important—than the nourishment and health of the blood and its circulatory system.

Weakened or stagnant qi is the precursor of disease. Disease itself, however, requires other factors, both internal and external, to take hold of the body. We shall consider these in the following chapter.

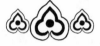

Chapter 2

THE CAUSES OF ILLNESS IN CHINESE MEDICAL THEORY

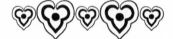

Chinese medical theory traditionally discerns three categories of causes of illness.[1] These are:

1. External factors, or *wai yin*. This classification encompasses climatic and environmental factors: wind, heat, fire, damp, dryness, and cold, as well as pestilence and epidemics.
2. Internal factors, or *nei yin*. This category includes both emotional disturbances that weaken the body's resistance to disease, and unhealthy behaviors such as prolonged malnutrition, overindulgence, inactivity, overstrain, and fatigue.
3. Neither external nor internal factors, or *bu nei bu wai yin*. Included in this category are injuries; wounds; parasites; insect, snake, and animal bites; and bacterial and viral infections.

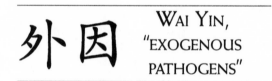

WAI YIN, "EXOGENOUS PATHOGENS"

The exogenous pathogens of traditional Chinese medical theory are sudden changes in the environment and climate due either to unseasonal aberrations in the weather or as a result of traveling from one region to another too quickly for the body to adapt. If the latter pathogenic factor was even considered in a time when the fastest means of transport was the horse (the Chinese were never much of a seafaring people), it must be reaching fairly epidemic proportions today as we hop around the planet, jumping several time zones and seasons in a matter of hours.

We are, without doubt, the most adaptable species living on this planet. Our ubiquitousness attests to that. Nevertheless, acclimatization takes time. Too sudden a change in the environment leads to imbalances. In Taoist terms, the Earth and the Water of places differ. The Five Elements within the body and the proportions of Yin and Yang change. *Zheng qi* ("proper" or "correct" qi, referring to the body's resistance to disease) is depleted in the effort to restore equilibrium. When qi is weak, illness is the likely outcome.

The climatic changes that are regarded as directly responsible for illness are collectively called the *xie qi*, or "evil qi."[2] They are evil wind (*feng*), cold (*han*), damp heat (*shu*), humidity (*shi*), intense dryness (*zao*), and firelike heat (*huo*). Although the xie qi are principally environmental, or external, factors affecting the body, the symptoms they produce frequently become manifest only when they enter to the very core of the body, affecting the zang and fu organs. When this happens they are considered xie qi syndromes of an internal nature.

風 Feng, "evil wind"

Evil wind is a Yang pathogenic factor. As such, it tends to attack the upper body (Yang) first. It is characterized by swift movement affecting various parts of the body in rapid succession, and by outward dispersion. It often operates in conjunction with another of the evil qi, giving rise to wind cold, wind heat, wind dampness, and, especially, wind fire. The latter is the most virulent combination, as wind is said to fan the Fire. The result is acute and persistent fever.

Common effects of a feng syndrome: The common cold, fevers, sweating, joint pains, itchy skin, spasms, and uncontrolled movements of the limbs. Wind tends to attack the liver. When it does, apoplexy, infantile convulsions, paralysis, and Parkinson's disease can result.

Early clinical manifestations: Headache, sore throat, blocked or runny nose, fever, perspiration, cough.

寒 Han, "cold"

Han, or cold, is a Yin pathogen. It depletes the Yang of the body, particularly that of blood and qi circulation. It is thus characterized by stagnation and by contracting of the blood vessels and muscles.

Common effects of a han syndrome: Aching muscles and joints, headache, cough, asthma, nasal blockage, pharyngitis. Sometimes a cold syndrome is brought about by the consumption of cold and uncooked food, or by exposure of the abdomen to cold. When this occurs cold tends to attack the spleen and stomach, thus affecting digestion. The effects are vomiting, diarrhea, and abdominal cramps.

Early clinical manifestations: Vomiting, stomachache, general feeling of cold in the extremities and in the abdomen.

暑 Shu, "summer heat"

Shu, or damp (summer) heat, is a Yang syndrome. It is said to consume Yin and qi. As with all Yang syndromes it affects the upper body, especially the head, giving rise to headaches, dizziness, and excessive sweating.

Common effects of a shu syndrome: Fever, heat sensation on the skin, irritability, rapid pulse, thirst, heavy head, stuffy chest, nausea and vomiting, abdominal distention, diarrhea.

Early clinical manifestations: Thirst, general weakness, yellow and scanty urine, constipation.

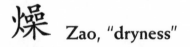 Shi, "damp"

Shi is a Yin pathogen. Its principal action is to obstruct the circulation of zheng qi, the body's disease-resistant force, resulting in sensations of heaviness, stagnation, and sluggishness. Shi usually attacks the lower half of the body (Yin), causing soreness in the muscles and joints of the lower limbs. It is also said to attack the spleen which, being of the Earth element, is particularly susceptible to humidity. The results are distention and soreness of the trunk and abdomen.

Common effects of a shi syndrome: Rheumatism, indigestion and constipation, skin rashes and fungi.

Early clinical manifestations: Lethargy in the head and body; aching in the limbs; fever; white, viscous-coated tongue; slow pulse.

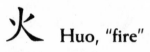 Zao, "dryness"

Zao, or dryness, is considered a Yang pathogen. It consumes Yin substance, especially body fluids. It tends to affect the chest, particularly the lungs, which need humidity to function adequately. Dryness may be either cold or hot, external or internal.

Common effects of a zao syndrome: Cold dryness results in symptoms similar to that of han, or cold, syndrome: aching muscles, joints, and head; cough; asthma; nasal blockage; pharyngitis further complicated by insufficient body fluid. Hot dryness causes headaches; a dry, rasping cough; thirst; irritability; red and dry mucous in the mouth and nose. Internal dryness is more serious than external; it can lead to mental instability and emotional distress.

Early clinical manifestations: Dry, rough skin and chapped lips.

火 Huo, "fire"

Huo, fire, is both one of the wu xing (Five Elements), and one of the six evil qi. It is a Yang pathogen that tends to flare upward. As a consequence, it consumes Yin fluids in the upper half of the body.

Common effects of a huo syndrome: Fever, thirst, heavy perspiration, ulcers of the tongue and mouth, nosebleed, irritability, anxiety, and insomnia. In extreme cases a fire syndrome can lead to delerium and loss of consciousness.

Early clinical manifestations: Thirst, dry mouth and throat, headache, red and swollen eyes, yellowish urine, dry stool, rapid heartbeat.

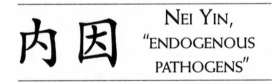 NEI YIN, "ENDOGENOUS PATHOGENS"

According to traditional Chinese medical theory the internal factors held responsible for the weakening of zheng qi, and hence the development of disease, are behavioral or emotional in nature. They are:

1. wrong eating habits
2. a stressful lifestyle
3. overindulgence in sex
4. the seven pathogenic emotions

Wrong Eating Habits

The pillar of good health is moderation in all things—exactly what parents always tell their children. Moderation—what amounts to common sense—in China became a working medical hypothesis. This hypothesis eventually became theory, and that theory led to a regimen adopted by every health-conscious individual in the country. In China we believe in the value of a long and healthy life. We therefore stick to moderation in whatever we do.

For most Chinese people, moderation means remembering, first of all, the "five forbiddens" (*wu jin*) of eating. They are:

1. Refrain from monotony. Do not eat only what appeals to your palate, but vary your diet at every meal.
2. Avoid excesses: eat spicy, sour, fried, salty, and sweet food sparingly.
3. Never eat large amounts at a single sitting. You should rise from the dinner table feeling only two-thirds full.
4. Beware of chemical additives and exotic foods. The latter refers to some Chinese delicacies, so infamous in the West, that we actually eat only as a special culinary adventure. These include snake meat, scorpion, insects, dog, badger, mouse, bear paws, snail, and turtle.
5. Do not overindulge in beverages in place of eating solid food.

In addition to these five forbiddens, Chinese medical tradition points out that overeating leads to stress on the digestive system, inefficient absorption of nutrients, weak qi, and disease. Malnutrition, on the other hand, deprives qi and blood of the nutrients necessary to life. Malnutrition includes eating too little for one's body weight; consuming a monotonous, poorly balanced diet; eating contaminated, poisonous, or stale food; and consuming cold food and drinks. Finally, overindulgence in intoxicating liquor is seen as a cause of serious imbalances and maladies, with the liver being particularly affected.

Stressful Lifestyle

In China we regard both overstrain and too little physical exertion as factors leading to imbalances and illness.

Overexertion over a long period weakens the body as a whole. It leads to exhaustion, dizziness, sleepiness, fluttering heart, asthma, and low resistance to disease.

Lack of physical exertion causes stagnation in the circulation of qi and blood to the various parts of the body. This results in unhealthy zang and fu organs, weakness, anorexia, dizziness, palpitations, insomnia, and a decreased resistance to the six evil qi exogenous pathogenic factors.

Overindulgence

Excessive sexual activity is considered to be a specific form of strain that consumes the kidney (water) essence and leads to lumbar pains, dizziness, ringing in the ears, listlessness, spermatorrhea, leukorrhea, and, in the long run, impotence in men and frigidity in women. What would be considered excessive sex is, perhaps, a matter of opinion; in China, engaging in sex more than twice a week is considered excessive.

The Seven Pathogenic Emotions

If a stressful lifestyle is considered deleterious to health, stressful emotions are seen as the pathogens that, one after another, get into your body, affect your qi and your internal organs, and, in the long run, lead to disease. So dangerous are they considered that Chinese medical tradition refers to them specifically as the seven pathogenic emotions. These are anger, melancholy, worry, grief, fear, fright, and joy.

The latter emotion may appear out of place—the experience of joy does not seem likely to lead to stress, distress, and a consequent lowering of resistance to disease. Nevertheless, we in China believe that when any of these emotions are too strong or constant, or when the subject is too sensitive to them, they cause imbalances within the body's zheng qi, and hence lead to disease. Anger is said to make the qi rush upward; joy makes it circulate slowly; grief consumes qi; fear causes it to flow downward; fright makes it flow unevenly; melancholy depletes qi; and worry leads to its stagnation.

A specific relationship is said to exist between each of the principal organ/Elements and the emotions (see table 1). It is recognized, therefore, that anger (Wood) injures the liver (also Wood). Melancholy and grief injure the lungs (Metal), fear injures the kidneys (Water), and joy injures the heart (Fire). It follows also that worry injures the spleen (Earth).

BU NEI BU WAI YIN, "NEITHER ENDOGENOUS NOR EXOGENOUS PATHOGENIC FACTORS"

This category includes wounds; injuries; insect, snake, and animal bites; parasites; fungi; and in our modern day, viruses and germs.

To deal with these factors, including germs and viruses, Chinese medicine resorts to foods and herbs that build qi and strengthen the body's resistance to disease. Nothing in ancient China was known about bacterial and viral infections. According to classical theory, however, no illness of any kind can enter or perpetuate itself within the body as long as qi is strong and circulates freely. As a result all therapies are aimed exclusively at helping the body defend itself, not at eliminating the external microscopic cause.

In practice this holistic approach works well with all ailments except the most virulent. This is the reason traditional Chinese medicine cannot deal with infections as successfully as modern allopathic (Western) medicine. Nevertheless, even today, when most city dwellers in China turn to allopathy for cures to maladies of a bacterial or viral nature, we invariably follow the dictates of traditional medicine at the same time. We may take antibiotics to cure the flu, but, with the antibiotics, we will take garlic and ginger broth with sugar for its warming effect, consume *yin qiao* pills to dispel fever, and crawl under a heavy quilt fully dressed for a good diaphoretic sweat.[3]

CHINESE THEORY AND THE WESTERN PARADIGM

The fact that Taoist theories of Yin and Yang, the Five Elements, and exogenous climatic pathogens do not fit current Western views of the world may be a matter of concern to many people. In the West, certain facts about nature and disease have been discovered that have opened avenues of therapy undreamed of just fifty years ago, and it would seem that any system of medicine that ignores these facts is bound to be deficient in one way or another. However, the two medical systems of allopathy and Chinese tradition are so different that any attempt to relate one to the other on theoretical grounds is futile. It would be rather like trying to compare the styles and techniques of traditional Peking opera with those of Western classical music, *wushu* boxing with a world heavyweight title bout, or qi gong with athletic training. The two systems simply arise from different traditions that view the world differently and have attributed different labels to reality as they see it.

It is possible, therefore, that traditional Chinese medical theory does not "ignore the facts" known to allopathy—it just looks at them from a different point of view. That point of view may have its own shortcomings, and we shall examine those in a moment. It may, however, also contain insights into humankind's relationship with nature that people who look at the world through Western eyes are still in the process of discovering.

The Western worldview is confident that disease is caused by exogenous pathogens with strange and exotic Greek and Latin names that can be isolated in laboratories and examined under microscopes. It is ascertained that if any of these exogenous pathogens enter the human body they will cause disease or, at the very least, cause an antipathogenic reaction as the body swings its defense mechanisms into urgent action. The outcome depends as much on the efficiency of the immune system as on the virulence of the external pathogen.

Chinese medicine asserts, on the other hand, that disease is caused by exogenous pathogens (with strange and exotic Chinese names) that twenty-five centuries ago were isolated as functions of nature and have been examined, ever since, in the field of human pathological experience. It is ascertained that if any of these exogenous

pathogens enter the body they will cause disease or bring about an antipathogenic reaction. The outcome depends as much on the state of internal health, or balance of all the elements of nature, as on the virulence of the external pathogen.

We do not wish to argue that the traditional Chinese doctors know as much about microbiology and biochemistry as any scientist in the West. They don't. Some of their ideas are worryingly old-fashioned and apparently impervious to change. What is more, a closed system used in a single country cannot hope to compete with the research going on worldwide, including in China, in all fields of allopathic medicine, microbiology, and genetics. Nonetheless, Chinese medicine does appear to consider aspects of biological nature that are still ignored in the West: our interconnectedness with the environment, for example; the importance of eating and living habits, which allopathic physicians often fail to notice; and the healthy management of the qi or vital energy, which we in China recognize as a universal force that circulates both within us and outside our bodies.

Fundamentally, allopathy tends to distinguish the human being from the causes of his or her disease, separate him or her from the environment, isolate the pathogen, and destroy it. Chinese medicine on the other hand considers causes of illness to arise from the interplay between the forces within the living human body and those in the environment. It does not isolate and destroy; instead, it purifies and strengthens.

The fact, therefore, that the West has been and continues to be in the midst of a dynamic process of discovery does not mean that we must throw out all that came before. As universal human beings we can maintain our skepticism, and our faith in the discoveries of Western medical science, while still benefiting from the ancient wisdom of traditional Chinese remedies.

Theories and strange names aside, traditional Chinese remedies can be seen to work. Ample evidence exists that they do. During the Tang dynasty (A.D. 618–907) an itinerant Chinese doctor named Sun Si Miao recommended the consumption of animal livers to cure night blindness. His assumption, tested by clinical practice, was that because the eyes and the liver are both of the Mu (Wood) Element function, a disease of the eyes could be corrected by strengthening the liver. He also believed, in common with Chinese tradition, that by consuming animal liver the patient's own liver would be nourished and strengthened.

It may be only a coincidence that Sun Si Miao's remedy worked, but work it did. We know today that night blindness is caused by a lack of vitamin A, and liver is a rich source of this vitamin. The consumption of liver will thus cure night blindness for reasons totally unknown during Sun Si Miao's lifetime, or indeed for many centuries after that.

Coincidence may have lain behind Sun Si Miao's remedies for goiter—caused by lack of iodine—which consisted of kelp, seaweed, and the thyroid glands of both lamb and pork, all of which are extremely rich in iodine. Similarly, his cure for beriberi—vitamin B_1 deficiency—consisting of taking vitamin B_1-rich rice bran and apricot seeds with milk, may have been quite fortuitous. On the other hand, the belief that food and drinks that induce perspiration can cure a cold, or that the consumption of energy-rich sugar and honey promote the reconstruction of the liver after a bout of infectious hepatitis, are both clinically and theoretically sound.

Consider, too, some of the discoveries of Chinese medicine:

❖ In the last century or two the people of the West have learned about the importance of hygiene and the value of disinfectants. In China we have known about them for two thousand years. The disinfectant properties of garlic, for example, have been recognized since the Han dynasty (206 B.C.–A.D. 220). Furthermore, Chinese people have throughout their entire history been aware of the dangers inherent in dirt, and have always been fastidious about cleanliness.

❖ In 1928 Alexander Fleming made what has been heralded as the greatest discovery of twentieth-century medical science: a mold, which he called penicillin, is an effective antibiotic, able to destroy many bacterial diseases. In China we have used molds and fungi against infections for at least 1340 years.[4]

❖ In nineteenth-century Europe it was discovered that a live virus low in virulence, when injected into a healthy person, will produce immunity in that person against the disease; the first vaccine to come into general use was that against smallpox. Chinese people have been vaccinating against smallpox since the Northern Song dynasty (960–1127), and perhaps even earlier.[5] The earliest technique was to grind some dried scabs taken from a smallpox patient and blow the powder into the nostril of the healthy person to be inoculated. Later, the technique was perfected; the juice of infected pus was transferred instead.[6]

❖ The first recorded case of the use of an amalgam of mercury for stopping and filling dental cavities was by Regnart, in Europe, in 1818. In China, silver paste was listed as a treatment for filling cavities in a materia medica of A.D. 659. A Ming dynasty materia medica from approximately A.D. 1500 actually specifies the ingredients used in Europe more than three hundred years later: One hundred parts of mercury to forty parts of silver and nine hundred parts of tin to form a paste that solidifies in the cavity.

There may be other examples that are still awaiting discovery by Western medical science.

Whether coincidental or not, forty-five hundred years of systematically recorded clinical practice have given the Chinese people one of the richest traditions of valid health directives and remedies of any country in the world. It is common sense to pay attention to it.

Chapter 3

EATING FOR HEALTH

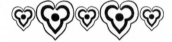

The Chinese concept of a balanced diet is different from Western concepts. It makes no mention of proteins, calories, vitamins, enzymes, and minerals. Instead, in China we refer to the flavors of foods, as well as to their qualities—the Yin/Yang and Five Element characteristics, and the food's nature as hot, warm, cool, or cold. Although the foundational tenets are different, in the end a balanced diet in both cultures amounts to the same thing: a varied regimen that ensures the consumption of moderate quantities of all available nutrients. The major difference in the two approaches is that the Chinese balanced diet takes into account not only the qualities of food but also those of the person eating it. The climate and the time of year are considered as well.

As a consequence of this wider approach one cannot make a straightforward assertion about whether any one food—mutton or coffee or spinach, for example—is good or bad for you. The value of any particular food is relative to your individual characteristics and the climatic conditions. If it is winter and you have a cold, Yin constitution, mutton and coffee are good for you. They have Yang and warming effects that counteract your personal nature and the climatic conditions. Spinach, on the other hand, is cool and may not be the ideal food for you in winter.

Before getting involved in more specifics regarding individual conditions and needs, let us look at some of the general do's and don'ts of Chinese preventive diet in regard to what and how, as well as when to eat.

❖ ❖ ❖

It is probably worth recalling the "five forbiddens" listed in chapter 2. These are:

1. Refrain from monotony. Do not eat only what appeals to your palate. Vary your diet at every meal.
2. Avoid excesses. Eat spicy, sour, fried, salty, and sweet food sparingly.
3. Never eat large amounts at a single sit-

ting. You should rise from the dinner table feeling only two-thirds full. Overeating leads to stress on the digestive system, inefficient absorption of nutrients, weak qi, and disease. Three light meals a day is the ideal. However, if you are very physically active and require more calories, several snacks through the day is better than one or two large meals.

4. Beware of exotic foods such as snake meat, scorpion, insects, bear paws, snails, and the like. These foods have their functions for some specific ailments but should not be eaten just for the sake of taste.

5. Do not overindulge in beverages instead of solid food. If you can do so comfortably, you should not drink at all during meals. The intake of liquids dilutes gastric juices and impairs digestion. Take your liquids before or after mealtimes.

Other rules are not even mentioned because they are simply common sense daily practices. These might be called the five *obvious* forbiddens. They are:

1. Do not eat too little for your body weight and energy expenditure.

2. Do not take toxic, contaminated, stale, rotting, or cold food or drinks.

3. Do not fry your food. If you must use oil, stir-fry briefly in a wok, or add a little raw oil to steamed or boiled food or to your salads.

4. Do not overcook your food. Overcooking destroys its heat-sensitive nutrients (enzymes and some vitamins).

5. Do not overindulge in alcoholic drinks. One beer, one glass of wine, or a single shot of spirits a day appears to have a positive effect on health. Anything more than this is poison.

Following the guidelines regarding what (and how) not to eat will in and of itself lead to better overall health. The customary Chinese way of eating is to serve small portions of many different foods. A traditional Western meal consisting of soup, steak, fried potatoes, and a dessert would be considered by the Chinese to be not only unhealthy but uncouth as well. First of all, there is not enough variety in the menu. Second, we believe that soup should come at the end of the meal (instead of a sweet dessert) in order to wash away strong flavors.[1] Third, most Chinese don't relish the idea of eating a slab of meat. We feel it cannot be cooked properly: either the outside is burned in order to cook the center, or else the inside is eaten raw—which for most Chinese people is too horrific even to contemplate. The only way we cook meat in China is to cut it into pieces. The origin of this practice was to save cooking fuel; however, it also ensures uniformity of cooking, as well as the possibility of sharing with others. Which brings us to our final point: eating individual portions is considered downright antisocial. And eating alone is abhorrent to most Chinese people: it is something that you do in a hurry, consuming perhaps your leftovers from a "real meal."[2] In China, people like to eat together; they like the hot and noisy atmosphere. And the more people there are, the more dishes and the more variety. The point, therefore, is to eat a little of a dozen or so food items at each sitting. A Chinese meal usually starts with a variety of cold dishes: boiled peanuts, ginger, raw tomato, cured jellyfish, bamboo tofu, germinated soybean shoots, and various cuts of cold meat. This is followed by alternating flavors and properties (warm, hot, cool, and cold) in the main dishes. Thus a dish of chicken (sweet [Earth] and warm) cooked with walnuts may be followed by spicy tofu (sweet [Earth] and cool) with hot and pungent [Metal] red pepper, by lettuce leaf in oyster sauce (cool and bittersweet [Fire and Earth]), and by shrimp with garlic (warm and sweet [Earth], balanced by the pungent (Metal) garlic—which, incidentally, also counteracts the cholesterol intake from the shrimp). The meal might proceed with green stringbeans, celery, and black mushrooms (all of which are sweet [Earth] and thermally neutral, with a dash of bitter [Fire] from the celery). If you had crab (cold and salty [Water]), you would eat it cooked with dry ginger (hot and pungent [Metal]) and vinegar (sour and bitter [Wood and Fire]) for balance. Finally, you would have either a bowl of rice or some steamed bread and a clear broth to wash it all down with.[3]

In China, everything is eaten: vegetables, fruits, seeds, roots, berries, fish, fowl, and all manner of four-legged creatures. A few purists argue that eating meat is harmful because it contaminates your vital energy with the grosser (that is, lesser refined) qi of animals; they, and Buddhist monks, are probably the only people in China who do not eat moderate quantities of meat fairly frequently. Yet meat is not the kind of health hazard in China that it is in the West. It is still seen as too much of a luxury to be overindulged in, and even those people who can afford it are aware of the dangers.[4]

Food should be consumed as soon after harvesting as possible, as some vitamins are dissipated in time. People in China make a point of shopping every day. Many families do not have refrigerators or freezers, and those who do possess a refrigerator do not keep food in it for more than a day. Indeed, the purpose of a refrigerator often has more to do with showing off one's new status symbol—or, for the more practically minded, for cooling drinks in summer—than with food preservation. Freezing destroys vitamin C, and canned food often consists of pure bulk, with no enzymes or vitamins. Canned food can also be contaminated by megadoses of preservatives and other toxins. For these reasons it is best to eat all foods as fresh as possible.

How to Eat

Moderation is the key not only to what you eat but to how you eat. The following guidelines should help you stay conservative in your intake.

- ❖ Eat only when you are hungry.
- ❖ Three meals a day are supposed to be most conducive to good health. Start with a large breakfast, follow it with a medium-sized lunch, and end the day with a light dinner at least three hours before bedtime. In China the evening meal is rarely taken much later than 7 P.M.
- ❖ Never eat when you are angry, upset, or in a state of emotional turmoil. Extreme emotions, considered to be one of the causes of disease, interfere with digestion.
- ❖ Eat slowly. Chopsticks elegantly used ensure that your food cannot be eaten too rapidly—by "elegantly used" we mean picking up each morsel and carrying it from your bowl to your lips.
- ❖ Chew your food properly and relish your drinks. Or, as the Chinese saying goes, "Drink your food and chew your drinks."
- ❖ Eat your food at room temperature if raw, or warm if cooked. Never eat food directly out of a refrigerator or piping hot. Extremes in heat and cold are a shock to the body.

- Do not talk when you eat. While people in China like to eat in large groups, they generally save their conversations for the time between courses.
- Eat in a warm and comfortable environment. Do not eat outdoors with your face into the wind; cold air is said to enter your body every time you open your mouth, causing stomachache.
- Avoid being sedentary immediately following a meal. A popular Chinese saying claims that "one hundred steps after meals assures ninety-nine years of life."

When to Eat Various Foods

Other than the actual foodstuffs, climate and time of year are perhaps the most important considerations for someone intent upon maintaining good health through conscientious eating habits.

According to traditional Taoist medical theory, one of the main causes of disease are the exogenous pathogens: the climatic aberrations of evil wind, excessive cold, heat, dampness, dryness, and firelike heat. These pathogens are believed to enter the body and cause havoc with one's equilibrium. The flow of zheng qi is affected, the internal organs are weakened, the individual's personal constitution is thrown out of skew, and illness is the likely outcome.

Because of the interdependence of all nature, the cold and heat that can attack a person from the outside also exist within each one of us as part of our individual constitution—we may be hot, cold, dry, damp, excessive, or deficient physical types. They also exert their influence as warming, heating, cooling, and cold characteristics of

everything we eat.

It follows therefore that, when in the depth of a cruel northern Chinese winter a person curls up on a warm *kang* and considers what to have for dinner, he does not think of salads, seafood, and watermelon, all of which are cold foods.[5] Hot ginger soup, warm chicken, chestnuts, and a dried peach are more likely choices. While this may sound like common sense, because anything and everything is available year-round in Western supermarkets people often make what, in Chinese eyes, would be considered very poor food choices given personal temperament and time of year.

It is important for one's health to eat according to season. Foods that are either slightly warming or cooling and those that are thermally neutral can be consumed without ill consequence during any season. Foods that exert powerful heating or cooling effects should not be consumed in the "wrong" season lest they exacerbate the influence of the pervading climate. However, taking cold food in summer will ensure greater resistance to summer heat. Hot foods in winter, on the other hand, protect against the cold.

Often, distinguishing between hot and cold foods is a matter of intuition or common sense. Nobody would consider black or white pepper cooling, nor would most people regard watermelon as warming. Often, however, we might be in doubt as to the thermal effects of bananas, crabs, or clams (all cold foods), or soybean oil (a hot food). We have therefore drawn up a list of cooling, cold, warming, and hot foods to help guide you in developing your awareness and making proper food choices. It is useful to remember that hot and warm thermal characteristics always correspond to Yang, and that cold and cool foods are always Yin.

Yin Foods

Cooling: apples, barley, tofu, mushrooms, cucumber, eggplant, zucchini, lettuce, lamb's liver, loquat, mandarin orange, mango, marjoram, mung bean, oyster shell, pear, peppermint, radish, sesame oil, spinach, strawberries, tangerine, wheat (and bran), fresh nonmatured coconut, yogurt, tea, jujube, rosehips.

Cold: bananas, grapefruit, melon, watermelon, persimmon, sugar cane, tomato, water chestnut, bamboo shoots, bitter gourd, lotus seed, egg white, clam, crab, kelp, seaweed, salt.

Yang Foods

Warming: apricot seed, asparagus, brown sugar, butter, caraway, fish, cherry, chestnut, chicken, chive, cinnamon twig, clove, mature coconut, coffee, coriander, cuttlefish, dates, orange, tangerine, grapefruit or mandarin peel, eel, fennel, garlic, fresh ginger, ginseng, green onion (scallion), guava, ham, kidney, liver, kumquat, mustard, leek, longan, lychee, malt, meat, milk, mussels, nutmeg, peaches, raspberries, rosemary, shrimp, spearmint, pumpkin, anise seed, sunflower seed, basil, rice, broad beans, vinegar, walnuts, wine, alcohol.

Hot: cinnamon bark, dried ginger, black or white pepper, red or green pepper, soybean oil, pork and greasy meats, cream, cocoa, chocolate, butter.

PERSONAL CONSTITUTION

Every individual has his or her personal characteristics in terms of body build, Yin and Yang, hot and cold, damp and dry, and excessive or deficient constitution. The relations and imbalances between these factors are wholly individual in nature. It therefore becomes important, when balancing your diet, to be aware of your personal characteristics so that abundant qualities are balanced and deficient qualities are enhanced.

A thin person of reddish complexion who prefers cold drinks and food to hot is generally considered to be a preponderantly hot (Yang) physical type. A plump person who is seldom thirsty and prefers hot drinks to cold is said to be of the cold, Yin type. Heavily built, lethargic people are damp (Yin) in character. Wiry individuals who are forever thirsty and suffer from dry skin, hair, nose, and mouth are considered dry (Yang).

The descriptives used to classify a person as hot or cold, damp or dry, deficient or excessive are similar to the classifications of the wai yin (external pathogenic) disease syndromes discussed in chapter 2. The same words are also used to describe the nature of various foods. Good health is seen as the balanced interplay between these properties in the environment, in the human body, and in food and drink. For example, the tall, thin person of ruddy complexion—the Yang, hot and dry characteristics mentioned above—will achieve optimum health by balancing his or her natural tendencies with Yin cold and lubricating foods, such as banana, grapefruit, orange, mango, pear, persimmon, strawberry, watermelon, lettuce, celery, tomato, seaweed, milk, honey, egg, and seafood (except shrimp). If, on the other hand, this person should eat large quantities of meat, scaly fish, or strong Yang foods that are spicy, hot, or salty, he would begin to suffer from lack of energy, indigestion, and eventually from imbalances that lead to illness.

The damp, heavily built person would do well to consume plenty of warm Yang foods: apricot, cherry, lemon, lychee, longan, papaya, raspberry, peach, chestnut, garlic, ginger, fennel, green onion (scallion), radish, peanut, potato, grains (brown rice and bread), beans, shrimp, and a little wine. Large quantities of dairy products, fats, and meat would increase the lethargy and convert into body fats.

Finding your personal body type is a multifaceted exploration. There are several factors to consider beyond build. These include your body heat, your moods and dispositions, your sex drive, and others. No person is exclusively one physical type. Furthermore, energy levels, moods, and the climate change all the time, affecting your physical condition. It would be ideal to consult a Chinese physician for a professional opinion regarding your overall Yin or Yang nature and whether your bodily constitution is essentially hot, cold, dry, humid, excessive, or deficient. However, self-observation aided by the following questionnaire should allow you to make a fairly precise assessment of your underlying physical characteristics.[6]

Personal Characteristics Questionnaire

Give yourself one point for each question you answer in the affirmative, two points if you feel that the question suits you particularly well.

Yin

If you are a woman, give yourself two Yin points.

Do you consider yourself feminine?

Are you timorous?

Are you the indoor type?

Do you tire easily?

Do you consider yourself lazy?

Do you fall asleep easily when traveling by plane, train, or bus?

Are your hands often cold?

Are your feet often cold?

Do you prefer the cold of winter to the heat of summer?

Are you overweight? (If you answer yes, score one point for every ten pounds over the normal weight for your sex and build.)

Is food better than or just as interesting as sex?

Do you consider your sex drive to be weaker than normal?
(Give yourself two points if you answer in the affirmative.)

Cold constitution

Do you rarely feel thirsty?

Do you generally prefer hot drinks to cold ones?

Is your complexion usually pale?

Is your urine normally plentiful and clear?

Are your stools normally soft?

Is your tongue usually pink with no coating?

Do you suffer from muscular or joint pains in cold weather?

Damp constitution

Do you often feel tired?

Are you overweight?

Is your complexion usually dull?

Are you often sad or depressed?

Do your palms sweat?

Is your tongue usually glossy or greasy?

Do your joints ache when it's raining?

Deficient constitution

Are you often low-spirited?

Are you often tired?

Are you skinny or underweight?

Do you sweat a lot?

Do you sometimes suffer from heart palpitations?

Are you of pale or pallid complexion?

Is your tongue white or light pink without coating?

YANG

If you are a man, give yourself two Yang points.

Do you consider yourself masculine?

Are you generally self-confident?

Are you the outdoor type?

Can you work for long stints without tiring?

Do you consider yourself energetic?

Do you find it difficult to sleep when traveling by plane, train, or bus?

Are your hands often hot?

Do your feet sweat?

Do you prefer the heat of summer to the cold of winter?

Are you underweight? (If your answer is yes, score one point for every ten pounds below the normal weight for your sex and build.)

Is sex better than food?

Do you consider your sex drive to be higher than normal?
  (Give yourself two points if you answer in the affirmative.)

Hot constitution

Do you normally prefer cold drinks to warm or hot ones?

Is your complexion generally reddish?

Is your urine usually scanty and of a reddish or yellow hue?

Are you often constipated?

Are your stools usually dry?

Is your tongue normally red with a yellowish coating or no coating?

Do you suffer from frequent skin eruptions?

Dry constitution

Are you often thirsty?

Are your nose, throat, and skin usually dry?

When you catch cold, is your cough usually dry without mucus?

Do your eyes and nose often itch?

Is your tongue frequently parched and dry?

Is it difficult for you to gain weight?

Are you often constipated?

Excessive constitution

Are you usually full of energy?

Do you consider yourself to be normally high-spirited?

Is the tone of your voice high-pitched?

Is your complexion usually flushed?

Is your blood pressure higher than normal?

Are you restless and impatient?

Do you suffer from constipation?

When you have completed the questionnaire, first add only your scores under the two main headings Yin and Yang; do not include your cold, damp, deficient, hot, dry, and excessive constitution scores in your first tally. The first total will tell you your predominant Yin/Yang characteristic. Few people are ever wholly Yin or Yang, so even if you are an energetic, self-confident male who enjoys sex and the outdoor life, it does not mean that you will have a score of 0 in the Yin section.

Now add up your bodily constitution scores. Once you have these tallied, add the cold, damp, and deficient numbers to your Yin scores; then add the hot, dry, and excessive numbers to your Yang scores. In the end, most people will find themselves scoring more or less equally on both Yin and Yang.

The point of this exercise is simply to be aware of your general tendencies. You will then be in a position to correct any imbalances in your constitution before they begin to affect your health. However, before you go about making drastic changes to your eating habits, you must first bring the Yin or Yang effects of climate into your calculations. If you have a 24 Yin score and a 17 Yang, for example, you might be tempted to include ginger, garlic, or onion in your diet for their warming effects. If it's the middle of summer, however, eating warming foods such as these would be a mistake—summer heat on its own counteracts any Yin or cold tendencies in your body. To further increase the heat with ginger and garlic would overbalance you in the opposite, Yang, direction.

In order to bring climatic effects into your personal Yin and Yang scores, add points according to the season, as shown in the following table.

TABLE 3: YIN AND YANG EFFECTS OF CLIMATE	
Spring	3 Yang points
Cool summer	5 Yang points
Hot summer	8 Yang points
End of summer (September, October)	0 points
Autumn	3 Yin points
Warm winter	5 Yin points
Cold winter	8 Yin points

If, in the final analysis, you find that your Yin and Yang or your body constitution scores are significantly different, all it means is that you should try to include a little more balancing food in your diet in proportion to the differences. Increase your intake of Yin or Yang, warm or cool foods by 10 percent for every five-point spread on the overall Yin/Yang scores. Try also to include more hot and warming foods in your diet if the questionnaire indicates you are of cold, damp, or deficient constitution, or if it is winter; conversely, eat a little more cold or cooling food if you are the hot, dry, or excessive physical type, or if it is summer.

❖ ❖ ❖

It should be clear by now that Chinese theories of health offer few simple do's and don'ts regarding diet. Health-giving food choices depend on personal constitution, the time of year, and the nature of disease a person might be suffering from. Only when you have a clear picture of your personal health needs can you choose your diet with confidence, noting the warming or cooling properties of foods, their taste and Element, and whether they lubricate or constrict. To help you in growing more discerning, the following chapter, Foods and Their Healing Properties, details the properties (in Chinese terms), vitamin and mineral contents, and usage of many foods commonly employed in Chinese therapeutic cuisine.

Chapter 4

FOODS AND THEIR
HEALING PROPERTIES

Traditionally, no clear-cut distinction is made between medicinal drugs, folk and home remedies, and many of the ingredients of classic Chinese cuisine. Garlic, cloves, and ginger, for example, are used in medicine, in folk remedies, and for cooking. Nevertheless, since antiquity medicinal drugs and ingredients have been classified into one of three possible categories of toxicity.

The first of the three categories is that of so-called high-grade drugs. These are wholesome beyond their purely medicinal function and can therefore be taken continuously over a period of time with no ill effects. Food therapies fit into this category. The second class is that of medium-grade drugs. These are slightly toxic but serve to relieve some deficiency syndromes. The third category is that of toxic, or low-grade, drugs. These may be taken in small doses for short periods of time, and only to relieve a specific disorder. Toxic herbs and mushrooms and some minerals fall into this class. Modern allopathic

drugs, if used by a traditional Chinese medic combining modern and ancient therapies, would also fit into this third category.[1]

Foods and drugs may be further defined for therapeutic purposes according to their Yin and Yang preponderances; their flavors, and thus their Five Element affinities; and their warm, hot, cool, and cold characteristics.

Yin and Yang are, in the Taoist view of the world, the most obvious attributes of nature. As such they are the first aspects of a patient's condition to attract a doctor's attention. The restoration of their equilibrium is the goal to which all therapy aims. As a consequence, foods and drugs that are considered to be of a Yin nature will be prescribed in disorders involving Yin deficiencies or Yang pathogens. Yang therapies serve to treat Yang deficiencies or Yin disorders.

Yin foods and remedies are those with moist, cool, or cold properties, for these are Yin characteristics. Yang foods, on the

35

other hand, have a warming or heating effect on the body. Yang remedies tend to exert most influence on the skin, tissues, and external parts of the body, while Yin remedies work on the internal organs. Yang foods and drugs ascend and disperse; those that are Yin in nature descend with an astringent effect. Yang foods and drugs are pungent, sweet, or tasteless. Yin remedies are sour, bitter, and salty.

Table 1 on page 11 shows the correspondence between the Five Elements in nature and various attributes of human physiology. One of those attributes is flavor. Each of the Elements/functions of nature is said to reside in one of the five flavors. Thus sour food, being of the Wood (germinating) element, influences the health of the liver, which is also Wood. Bitterness corresponds to Fire and affects the heart; sweetness to Earth and spleen. Pungent foods, those of the Metal element, affect the lungs; salty foods correspond to Water and influence the health of the kidneys. It is believed that by taking foods with a specific flavor/Element, the corresponding organ of the body is strengthened. Furthermore, each of the five flavors is said to exert its own therapeutic effect on the body as a whole. We shall therefore refer to the flavor, the Element, and the effect of the foods examined later in this chapter.

As a matter of interest, the effects of sour foods and drugs are said to be astringent; they counteract digestive problems and diarrhea. Bitter ingredients are febrifuges; in other words, they dispel fevers. Sweet foods act as a tonic to the body. Pungent, or tangy, ingredients act as diaphoretics; they induce sweat, reduce intestinal and stomach gas, and are said to promote the movement of qi within the body. Salty ingredients are palliatives, which means they reduce excesses and imbalances of the Five Elements as well as the effects of pathogens. Tasteless foods are considered to be diuretics.

Finally, a word about the so-called warming and cooling characteristics of foods and drugs. Illness, according to Chinese theory, is frequently brought about by the effects of the six evil climatic factors, the xie qi: evil wind, cold, damp heat, humidity, intense dryness, and firelike heat. If, as according to this theory, cold enters the body and causes disease, it is simply common sense to counteract it with warm or hot ingredients. Similarly, cool or cold foods and drugs are used to disperse hot climatic pathogens. The terms *warm, hot, cool, cold,* and *neutral* may, however, be confusing. They do not refer to the actual physical temperature of the remedy being taken, but instead denote a fundamental property of the food or ingredient after it has been swallowed and digested. A steaming cup of tea, for example, may exert an immediate warming effect on the body, but tea is fundamentally a "cold" herb, useful for cooling the body (and, incidentally, for burning fats and promoting digestion).

Having mentioned these classifications, it should be noted that few foods or ingredients ever fit a single and precise category—Yin always contains some Yang and vice versa. Herbs, fruits, and vegetables usually combine several distinct flavors. Tea (*Camellia sinensis*), in both its black and green varieties, is sweet, bitter, and pungent at the same time. Peaches are both sweet and sour. Asparagus is bitter and slightly pungent. A single food item, therefore, may potentially have several therapeutic effects.

A final word about how ingredients can and cannot be used is perhaps called for before continuing on to examine the foods and components of Chinese remedies themselves.

Sometimes a single product, such as ginseng, can be used alone to treat an illness. On other occasions ingredients are combined in order to exert a fuller curative effect on the patient—food recipes are a case in point. These combinations are not always straightforward, however. Sometimes two ingredients mutually reinforce each other; on other occasions a subsidiary ingredient will assist the function of the other, principal component. There are situations also when one Element is necessary to restrain the toxic effect of another. Finally, some ingredients are so incompatible as to give rise to severe side effects if used together.

As an illustration of this last point of incompatibility, ingredients with warm properties acting on the lungs should never be taken with raw and cold (temperature-wise) food. Cooling ingredients should not be taken with greasy foods. Meat should be eaten sparingly when taking black plum for therapeutic reasons. Turnips, radishes, and rape should not be eaten when one takes tonics; neither should black or green tea. Both are said to weaken the strengthening power of the tonic.[2]

Apart from refraining from drinking tea with tonics, there is no need for you to concern yourself about any of the above combinations and contraindications. All the remedies described in this book have been chosen for their simplicity and straightforward wholesomeness. Unless one happens to be allergic to any of the ingredients, none of the recipes will exert the least adverse effect. As to the means and methods of preparation of various prescriptions used in popular Chinese remedies, we refer you to chapters 5 and 6.

❖ ❖ ❖

Let us now look at the characteristics of the individual foods and herbs used in the Chinese home remedies described in this book. For the purpose of self-diagnosis and gentle experimentation with individual foods, we have given the characteristics of each ingredient in Chinese terms—sweet/sour and corresponding Element, hot/cold, Yin/Yang—as well as in Western terms—protein, fat, carbohydrate, mineral, and vitamin contents per 100 grams ($3\frac{1}{2}$ ounces) of edible portion.[3] A mineral or vitamin that is completely absent will be denoted by a zero; a minus sign denotes that the information for that particular nutrient is unavailable. (See appendix 1 for information on daily requirements of those vitamins and minerals for the healthy adult.) In addition to this information, we discuss the predominant healing effects of that food. Most of the foods discussed in this chapter are commonly available in the market; a few will be found in specialty food stores or by mail order. Sources for mail order are given in appendix 2.

FRUITS

Fruits are some of the most nutritious foods available to us. They are rich in vitamins, minerals, enzymes, and fiber.

According to Chinese theory, fruit lubricates, cools, and strengthens the body. It is easily digested and cleanses the intestines. Most fruit is sweet, and therefore tonifies the Earth element.

It is preferable to consume fruit directly from the producer before various intermediaries have sprayed, artificially ripened, waxed, or otherwise adulterated it. Indeed, in China this is the norm. Most of the fruit that is consumed in China is produced locally, ripened on the tree or vine and eaten only in season.

Many fruits have a cooling, or even a cold, effect on the body. Banana, grapefruit, muskmelon, persimmon, and watermelon are all cold fruits. As such they are extremely refreshing during summer, but their consumption in winter could lead to cold-syndrome diseases. The traditional Chinese calendar even specifies a day in the second week of August, for eating one's last watermelon of the year.

It is best to eat organically grown fruit whenever possible. Most people are aware of the harmful effects of insecticides, and make a point of peeling fruit. However, peeling apricots, plums, strawberries, or grapes is not easy; furthermore, although chemicals are only sprayed on the outside of the fruit, they eventually seep through the entire plant. Organically grown produce of all kinds is becoming widely available. Look for it in natural foods markets.

Apple
Sweet and sour (Earth and Wood), cool, medium Yin

Apple aids digestion, lubricates the lungs, and generally detoxifies. It cures indigestion, morning sickness, and chronic enteritis, and combats diabetes by helping to lower blood-sugar levels. Its plentiful fiber helps to lower cholesterol, and its potassium content has a diuretic effect that reduces sodium and stabilizes blood pressure. Many of the nutrients reside in the skin of the apple; it is thus advisable to eat apples unpeeled—given, of course, that they have not been treated chemically.

Protein, 0.2 g; Fat, 0.3 g; Fiber, 1.4 g; Carbohydrate, 10.5 g; Vitamin A, 37 IU; Vitamin B₁, 0.01 mg; Vitamin B₂, 0.01 mg; Niacin, 0.05 mg; Vitamin C, 4 mg; Calcium, 5 mg; Phosphorus, 5 mg; Iron, 0.12 mg

Apricot
Sour and sweet (Wood and Earth), warm, neutral Yin/Yang

Apricot lubricates and strengthens the lungs; it alleviates asthma and dryness of the mouth. Apricot seeds are used in a variety of remedies. They are, however, considered a medium-grade drug in China. This means that they are slightly toxic, and should therefore only be taken in small quantities and for short periods of time. Bitter apricot seeds can suppress coughing, and are a valid relief for asthma.

Protein, 1 g; Fat, 0.1 g; Fiber, 0.6 g; Carbohydrate, 12.9 g; Vitamin A, 2790 IU; Vitamin B₁, 0.03 mg; Vitamin B₂, 0.05 mg; Niacin, 0.8 mg; Vitamin C, 7 mg; Calcium, 16 mg; Phosphorus, 23 mg; Iron, 0.5 mg

Banana
Sweet (Earth), cold, medium Yin

Banana has a lubricating effect on the intestines. It detoxifies the body by providing plenty of soluble fiber that absorbs cholesterol and cleanses the intestines. It cures constipation, hemorrhoids, and high blood pressure, and counteracts indigestion and alcoholism. Eat two soft bananas every morning to relieve constipation. Two ripe (but not soft) bananas stop diarrhea. The banana's high fiber content helps to lower blood cholesterol. A banana a day cures chronic indigestion. Eat cooked green bananas if you suffer from diabetes—the starch has not yet been converted into sugar.

Protein, 1.2 g; Fat, 0.6 g; Fiber, 1.6 g; Carbohydrate, 26.7 g; Vitamin A, 92 IU; Vitamin B₁, 0.05 mg; Vitamin B₂, 0.11 mg; Niacin, 0.6 mg; Vitamin C, 10 mg; Calcium, 7 mg; Phosphorus, 22 mg; Iron, 0.35 mg

Cherry
Sweet (Earth), warm, Yang

Cherries tone the qi and the blood, and counteract rheumatic pains and stiffness. They also expel wind and damp.

Protein, 1.1 g; Fat, 0.5 g; Fiber, 0.7 g; Carbohydrate, 14.8 g; Vitamin A, 620 IU; Vitamin B$_1$, 0.05 mg; Vitamin B$_2$, 0.06 mg; Niacin, 0.3 mg; Vitamin C, 8 mg; Calcium, 18 mg; Phosphorus, 20 mg; Iron, 0.4 mg

Fig
Sweet (Earth), neutral, Yang

Figs tonify the qi and blood. Because they clear the intestines, figs are a useful remedy for constipation and hemorrhoids. Chinese doctors also prescribe figs for sore throat and stomach and intestinal problems, including dysentery and diarrhea: eat two figs a day, either in the morning or in the evening. For a sore throat, steam them and take with honey.

Protein, 0.8 g; Fat, 0.4 g; Fiber, –; Carbohydrate, 19.2 g; Vitamin A, 140 IU; Vitamin B$_1$, 0.06 mg; Vitamin B$_2$, 0.06 mg; Niacin, 0.4 mg; Vitamin C, 2 mg; Calcium, 32 mg; Phosphorus, 14 mg; Iron, 0.32 mg

Grapes
Sweet and sour (Earth and Wood), neutral, balance of Yin and Yang

Grapes are a great builder of red blood cells. They have been used since antiquity to tonify the blood and qi. They are eaten as a general tonic as well as to treat coughs, promote urination, and relieve dryness and thirst.

American Concord grapes: Protein, 1.4 g; Fat, 1.4 g; Fiber, 0.5 g; Carbohydrate, 14.9 g; Vitamin A, 80 IU; Vitamin B$_1$, 0.06 mg; Vitamin B$_2$, 0.04 mg; Niacin, –; Vitamin C, 4 mg; Calcium, 17 mg; Phosphorus, 21 mg; Iron, 0.6 mg

European adherent skin grapes: Protein, 0.8 g; Fat, 0.4 g; Fiber, 0.5 g; Carbohydrate, 16.7 g; Vitamin A, 80 IU; Vitamin B$_1$, 0.06 mg; Vitamin B$_2$, 0.04 mg; Niacin, –; Vitamin C, 4 mg; Calcium, 17 mg; Phosphorus, 21 mg; Iron, 0.6 mg

Grapefruit
Sweet and sour (Earth and Wood), cool, medium Yin

Grapefruit aids digestion and stimulates the appetite. By virtue of its cooling characteristics, grapefruit can reduce fevers and eliminate toxins. It is especially useful for overcoming intoxication from alcohol.

Protein, 0.5 g; Fat, 0.2 g; Fiber, 0.3 g; Carbohydrate, 10.1 g; Vitamin A, 12 IU; Vitamin B$_1$, 0.04 mg; Vitamin B$_2$, 0.02 mg; Niacin, –; Vitamin C, 40 mg; Calcium, 22 mg; Phosphorus, 18 mg; Iron, 0.7 mg

Guava
Sweet and sour (Earth and Wood), warm, Yang

Guava is regarded as having obstructive and constrictive effects on the metabolic processes. As a consequence, when taken raw or as a decoction it is a valid remedy for diarrhea and dysentery. Make a decoction to soothe a sore throat.

Protein, 0.6 g; Fat, 0.6 g; Fiber, 5.5 g; Carbohydrate, 17.1 g; Vitamin A, 250 IU; Vitamin B$_1$, 0.07 mg; Vitamin B$_2$, 0.04 mg; Niacin, 1.1 mg; Vitamin C, 302 mg; Calcium, 18 mg; Phosphorus, 29 mg; Iron, 0.7 mg

Jujube (Chinese date)
Sweet (Earth), warm, Yang

Jujube are one of our five most prized remedies in China; they have been grown as a medicinal fruit tree for at least four thousand years. The principal effect of jujube is to nourish the qi and blood, and strengthen the stomach and the body as a whole. Jujube are considered to maintain youthfulness. One traditional story tells of a woman who lived two thousand years ago who ate nothing but jujube. It is said that when she married, at the age of fifty, her appearance was that of a twenty-year-old virgin. To this day many women in China make a point of eating ten to twenty jujube every morning for the complexion.

As a tonic, jujube are usually prepared in decoctions or stews. One remedy for convalescents is to decoct 10 jujube with 10 grams of ginseng every morning. Another, for pregnancy and for a rapid recovery after childbirth, consists of 20 jujube, 2 tablespoons of brown sugar, and 1 egg stewed and eaten once a day.

Recent research in China has demonstrated that jujube has an antibiotic effect that increases the body's resistance to infection and disease.

Fresh: Protein, 1.2 g; Fat, 0.2 g; Fiber, –; Carbohydrate, 20.2 g; Vitamin A, 40 IU; Vitamin B$_1$, 0.02 mg; Vitamin B$_2$, 0.04 mg; Niacin, 0.9 mg; Vitamin C, 69 mg; Calcium, 21 mg; Phosphorus, 23 mg; Iron, 0.48 mg

Dried: Protein, 3.7 g; Fat, 1.1 g; Fiber, –; Carbohydrate, 73.6 g; Vitamin A, 95 IU; Vitamin B$_1$, 0.21 mg; Vitamin B$_2$, 0.36 mg; Niacin, 0.5 mg; Vitamin C, 13 mg; Calcium, 79 mg; Phosphorus, 100 mg; Iron, 1.8 mg

Lemon
Sour (Wood), neutral, Yang

Lemon is not common in China and is therefore not used extensively as a treatment. It is known to relieve nausea and dryness. Steamed lemon with sugar relieves coughing and catarrh. As a mouthwash, lemon juice helps guard against gum disease and will alleviate a sore throat. Lemon should *not* be taken by people suffering from acidity and ulcers.

Protein, 0.9 g; Fat, 0.2 g; Fiber, 0.9 g; Carbohydrate, 8.7 g; Vitamin A, 0 IU; Vitamin B$_1$, 0.04 mg; Vitamin B$_2$, 0.01 mg; Niacin, 0.6 mg; Vitamin C, 27 mg; Calcium, 40 mg; Phosphorus, 22 mg; Iron, 0.6 mg

Longan
Sweet (Earth), warm, Yang

Longan is a fruit that grows only in tropical climates. It is delicious fresh but may also be taken dried for medicinal purposes. It energizes qi; nourishes the blood, heart, and spleen; and expels cold. It is often prescribed for general debility, insomnia, and nervous disorders.

Protein, 1.0 g; Fat, 0.6 g; Fiber, 1.4 g; Carbohydrate, 15 g; Vitamin A, 200 IU; Vitamin B$_1$, 0.03 mg; Vitamin B$_2$, 0.07 mg; Niacin, –; Vitamin C, 24 mg; Calcium, 35 mg; Phosphorus, 19 mg; Iron, 1.2 mg

Lychee
Sweet (Earth), warm, balance of Yin and Yang

Lychee nourishes the qi and the blood and expels cold. It is sometimes used as an analgesic for toothache, and is often taken to halt a stubborn hiccup. Lychee alleviates stomachache and thirst. Steamed lychees are recommended as a cure for asthma.

Protein, 0.8 g; Fat, 0.4 g; Fiber, –; Carbohydrate, 16.5 g; Vitamin A, 0 IU; Vitamin B$_1$, 0.01 mg; Vitamin B$_2$, 0.07 mg; Niacin, 0.6 mg; Vitamin C, 72 mg; Calcium, 5 mg; Phosphorus, 31 mg; Iron, 0.31 mg

Mango
Sweet and sour (Earth and Wood), cool, balance of Yin and Yang

Mango nourishes qi, the blood, and the functions of the stomach. Its cooling effect dissipates hot-syndrome diseases. Mango is used to relieve nausea and vomiting, coughing, and weakness in the lungs and bronchi.

Protein, 0.55 g; Fat, 0.3 g; Fiber, 1.1 g; Carbohydrate, 17.6 g; Vitamin A, 4030 IU; Vitamin B$_1$, 0.06 mg; Vitamin B$_2$, 0.06 mg; Niacin, 0.6 mg; Vitamin C, 28 mg; Calcium, 11 mg; Phosphorus, 11 mg; Iron, 0.15 mg

Melon
Sweet (Earth), cold, Yin

Melon tones the qi and the blood. Its cold characteristic relieves the heat of summer. It is used as a diuretic.

Protein, 0.5 g; Fat, 0 g; Fiber, 0.4 g; Carbohydrate, 8.5 g; Vitamin A, 40 IU; Vitamin B$_1$, 0.05 mg; Vitamin B$_2$, 0.03 mg; Niacin, –; Vitamin C, 23 mg; Calcium, 17 mg; Phosphorus, 16 mg; Iron, 0.4 mg

Orange peel
Pungent and slightly bitter (Metal and Fire), warm, Yin

Orange peel affects the stomach and the internal organs of digestion. A decoction of orange peel and ginger will relieve gastritis. Orange peel brewed in water is a valid remedy for inebriation and a preventive against hangover. Dispersed in water, orange peel will also relieve coughs and chest catarrh.

Protein, 0.6 g; Fat, 0 g; Fiber, –; Carbohydrate, 10 g; Vitamin A, 165 IU; Vitamin B$_1$, 0.06 mg; Vitamin B$_2$, 0.06 mg; Niacin, 0.7 mg; Vitamin C, 53 mg; Calcium, 65 mg; Phosphorus, 7 mg; Iron, 0.33 mg

Papaya
Sweet (Earth), neutral, mild Yang

Papaya promotes digestion. It cures stomachache, dysentery, and difficult bowel movements. Because papaya dissipates dampness, it is a useful remedy for diseases of a damp nature, such as rheumatism and arthritis. A teaspoon of papaya seeds helps to detoxify the liver.

Fresh raw papaya is a good supplement to meals, in order to counteract indigestion.

Protein, 0.95 g; Fat, 0.2 g; Fiber, 1.4 g; Carbohydrate, 18.9 g; Vitamin A, 3061 IU; Vitamin B$_1$, 0.04 mg; Vitamin B$_2$, 0.05 mg; Niacin, 0.5 mg; Vitamin C, 94 mg; Calcium, 36 mg; Phosphorus, 8 mg; Iron, 0.15 mg

Peach
Sweet and sour (Earth and Wood), warm, mild Yang

Peaches are native to China. In Chinese mythology peaches represent immortality. According to legend, a peach tree that stands in the Kunlun mountains blossoms and bears fruit every nine thousand years. Whoever eats these peaches obtains immortal life.

Ordinary peaches, on the other hand, merely nourish the blood and qi, dissipate cold, and lubricate the intestines. Steamed peaches with a tablespoon of sugar or honey alleviates asthma and a bad cough. Fresh peaches are frequently taken as a remedy against high blood pressure.

Protein, 0.5 g; Fat, 0.1 g; Fiber, 0.6 g; Carbohydrate, 12 g; Vitamin A, 880 IU; Vitamin B$_1$, 0.02 mg; Vitamin B$_2$, 0.05 mg; Niacin, –; Vitamin C, 8 mg; Calcium, 8 mg; Phosphorus, 22 mg; Iron, 0.6 mg

Pear
Sweet and sour (Earth and Wood), cool, medium Yin

Pear affects the stomach and lungs. It lubricates, counteracting dryness, and is said to eliminate mucus. Fresh pear juice is drunk in China to relieve stubborn coughs and fever. Chinese pears are generally harder, juicier, and more sour than the American variety.

A curious superstition exists in China concerning pears. The word for pear, *li,* is pronounced exactly like another word meaning "separation." Many people therefore refuse to share a pear with a loved one for fear of bringing bad luck to their union.

Protein, 0.6 g; Fat, 0.5 g; Fiber, 4 g; Carbohydrate, 11.9 g; Vitamin A, 28 IU; Vitamin B$_1$, 0.06 mg; Vitamin B$_2$, 0.03 mg; Niacin, 0.02 mg; Vitamin C, 7 mg; Calcium, 8 mg; Phosphorus, 15 mg; Iron, 0.5 mg

Persimmon
Sweet (Earth), cold, medium Yin

The high tannic acid content of unripe persimmon has an "obstructive" or astringent consequence, making unripe persimmon effective in treating diarrhea, dysentery, and chest mucus.

When persimmon ripens, the tannic acid is converted into fructose. Ripe persimmon lubricates the lungs and nourishes the heart, spleen, and intestines. It relieves stomachache, hemorrhoids, and constipation. Persimmon is also used for regulating high blood pressure, treating canker sores in the mouth, and calming a stubborn cough.

Protein, 0.2 g; Fat, 0.1 g; Fiber, –; Carbohydrate, 8.4 g; Vitamin A, –; Vitamin B$_1$, –; Vitamin B$_2$, –; Niacin, –; Vitamin C, 17 mg; Calcium, 7 mg; Phosphorus, 7 mg; Iron, 0.63 mg

Pineapple
Sweet and sour (Earth and Wood), neutral, Yang

Pineapple should always be consumed ripe—underripe pineapple is acidic to the extreme and can cause stomach cramps and damage to the teeth and bones.

Soft, sweet pineapple, on the other hand, promotes digestion. It also promotes urination, quenches thirst, and heals swelling. Sweet pineapple stimulates the appetite and is therefore used to treat anorexia.

Protein, 0.6 g; Fat, 0.7 g; Fiber, 2.4 g; Carbohydrate, 19.2 g; Vitamin A, 35 IU; Vitamin B$_1$, 0.14 mg; Vitamin B$_2$, 0.06 mg; Niacin, 0.07 mg; Vitamin C, 24 mg; Calcium, 11 mg; Phosphorus, 11 mg; Iron, 0.57 mg

Plum
Sweet and sour (Earth and Wood), neutral, balance of Yin and Yang

Plum nourishes the blood and qi; it also combats dryness. In China plum is eaten to promote digestion and urination and to nourish weak kidneys or liver. A specific remedy for kidney or liver problems is a tea prepared from two crushed whole plums (including the seed) mixed with hot water and drunk twice a day.

Two plums soaked in vinegar and then boiled in water help cure canker sores, sore throat, and chronic tonsillitis. Use the cooled water for washing the mouth and for gargling.

Protein, 0.7 g; Fat, 0.2 g; Fiber, 0.5 g; Carbohydrate, 12.9 g; Vitamin A, 350 IU; Vitamin B$_1$, 0.06 mg; Vitamin B$_2$, 0.04 mg; Niacin, –; Vitamin C, 5 mg; Calcium, 17 mg; Phosphorus, 20 mg; Iron, 0.5 mg

Strawberry
Sweet and sour (Earth and Wood), cool, mild Yin

Strawberries nourish qi and lubricate the lungs. Because they are rich in vitamin C, silicon, and water, they alleviate thirst, generate body fluids, and have an antioxidizing effect on cells, blood vessels, and tissues. They also, as a consequence, flush out toxins and regulate urination and kidney function.

Eaten regularly with sugar, strawberries will cure a stubborn dry cough. As an appetizer, strawberries will stimulate the appetite and ensure good digestion. Strawberries are not native to China and have only been cultivated there recently. For this reason they do not figure prominently in Chinese medicine.

Protein, 0.8 g; Fat, 0.5 g; Fiber, 1.4 g; Carbohydrate, 8.3 g; Vitamin A, 60 IU; Vitamin B$_1$, 0.03 mg; Vitamin B$_2$, 0.07 mg; Niacin, –; Vitamin C, 60 mg; Calcium, 28 mg; Phosphorus, 27 mg; Iron, 0.8 mg

Tangerine
Sweet and sour (Earth and Wood), cool, mild Yin

Tangerine dissipates heat and dryness. It is often used for treating nausea, vomiting, hiccups, and catarrh in the chest. It is also useful in the treatment of diabetes.

Protein, 0.8 g; Fat, 0.3 g; Fiber, 1 g; Carbohydrate, 10.9 g; Vitamin A, 420 IU; Vitamin B$_1$, 0.07 mg; Vitamin B$_2$, 0.03 mg; Niacin, –; Vitamin C, 31 mg; Calcium, 33 mg; Phosphorus, 23 mg; Iron, 0.4 mg

Watermelon
Sweet (Earth), cold, mild Yin

The watermelon is native to Africa but has been cultivated in Asia for at least four thousand years. Because of its thirst-quenching and refreshing properties, watermelon is one of the most popular fruits in China during the hot summer.

Watermelon is a strong diuretic. It dissipates hot- and dry-syndrome problems, such as headaches, dry mouth and throat, red and dry mucus in the mouth and nose, red and swollen eyes, dry stool, rapid heartbeat, and irritability. It heals canker sores in the mouth and sore throat. Watermelon is useful for treating hangover. The rind and seeds are used to treat hypertension. A decoction using the seeds will also relieve constipation.

Protein, 0.5 g; Fat, 0.2 g; Fiber, 0.6 g; Carbohydrate, 6.9 g; Vitamin A, 590 IU; Vitamin B$_1$, 0.05 mg; Vitamin B$_2$, 0.05 mg; Niacin, –; Vitamin C, 6 mg; Calcium, 7 mg; Phosphorus, 12 mg; Iron, 0.2 mg

VEGETABLES

Vegetables constitute the second tier of the human food pyramid. As such, they are the second most important food source, following grains.

Vegetables contain vitamins, minerals, enzymes, and fiber. Enzymes both nourish and cleanse, while fiber absorbs toxins and cholesterol. Because of these properties, vegetables are particularly effective in detoxifyng the body. Ideally, four or five different vegetables should be eaten each day. Most vegetables should be eaten raw so as not to harm their enzyme and heat-sensitive vitamin contents. However, many vegetables are not easy to digest, and others, like carrots, require some cooking before the body is able to absorb their rich nutrient content. Frozen, canned, dried, or otherwise preserved vegetables lack the nutrient properties of fresh produce. Just as with fruit, vegetables are best consumed in season, and obtained from local organic sources.

Asparagus
Sweet and bitter (Earth and Fire), cold, mild Yin

Asparagus tones qi and dissipates heat and damp from the body. Its cold properties counteract fire-syndrome diseases, but render asparagus unsuitable in cold weather and when suffering from cold stomachache, diarrhea, or coughing. In China asparagus is prescribed as a diuretic. It is also useful in the treatment of diabetes and chronic bronchitis.

Protein, 2.2 g; Fat, 0.2 g; Fiber, 0.7 g; Carbohydrate, 3.9 g; Vitamin A, 1000 IU; Vitamin B$_1$, 0.16 mg; Vitamin B$_2$, 0.19 mg; Niacin, –; Vitamin C, 33 mg; Calcium, 21 mg; Phosphorus, 62 mg; Iron, 0.9 mg

Bamboo shoot
Sweet (Earth), cool, mild Yin

Bamboo shoot nourishes the blood and qi. Its cooling effect dissipates internal heat.

Bamboo shoot is used extensively in Chinese cuisine. The cooling effects of bamboo shoot balance the warming effects of meat. Its high fiber content is effective in treating constipation and in lowering cholesterol levels in the blood.

Protein, 2.0 g; Fat, 0.2 g; Fiber, 2.0 g; Carbohydrate, 4.0 g; Vitamin A, 15 IU; Vitamin B_1, 0.11 mg; Vitamin B_2, 0.05 mg; Niacin, 0.5 mg; Vitamin C, 3 mg; Calcium, 10 mg; Phosphorus, 45 mg; Iron, 0.38 mg

Carrot
Sweet (Earth), neutral, Yang

Carrot exerts a stimulating effect on digestion and nourishes the spleen. It is famed for improving night vision because of its vitamin A content.

Carrots are used in China for treating whooping cough. They are believed to play an important role in maintaining youthful skin and hair. Carrot juice is a valid remedy for anemia, and crushed raw carrot alleviates burns. However, carrots' nutrients are difficult to absorb when eaten raw. It is often preferable, therefore, to render them more easily digestible through cooking.

Protein, 0.7 g; Fat, 0.1 g; Fiber, 1.1 g; Carbohydrate, 7.3 g; Vitamin A, 20,253 IU; Vitamin B_1, 0.07 mg; Vitamin B_2, 0.04 mg; Niacin, 0.7 mg; Vitamin C, 7 mg; Calcium, 19 mg; Phosphorus, 32 mg; Iron, 0.36 mg

Celery
Sweet, pungent, and bitter (Earth, Metal, and Fire), cool, slightly Yin

Celery, a cooling food, eliminates dampness and nourishes and soothes the liver. Celery is one of the best food remedies for lowering high blood pressure. It also improves the texture of the hair and skin. Celery is traditionally used to treat whooping cough.

Protein, 0.3 g; Fat, 0.1 g; Fiber, 0.4 g; Carbohydrate, 1.5 g; Vitamin A, 51 IU; Vitamin B_1, 0.01 mg; Vitamin B_2, 0.01 mg; Niacin, 0.1 mg; Vitamin C, 3 mg; Calcium, 14 mg; Phosphorus, 10 mg; Iron, 0.19 mg

Chinese cabbage
Sweet (Earth), slightly cold, Yang

Chinese cabbage is a diuretic. It facilitates digestion and exerts a stimulating effect on the stomach and intestines. Chinese cabbage combats inflamation due to heat and Fire, such as rashes, redness and irritation of the eyes, sore throat, and constipation.

Protein, 0.5 g; Fat, 0.1 g; Fiber, –; Carbohydrate, 0.8 g; Vitamin A, 1050 IU; Vitamin B_1, 0.01 mg; Vitamin B_2, 0.03 mg; Niacin, 0.2 mg; Vitamin C, 16 mg; Calcium, 37 mg; Phosphorus, 13 mg; Iron, 0.28 mg

Cucumber
Sweet (Earth), cold, balance of Yin and Yang

Cucumber cleans the blood and detoxifies by promoting urination. It affects the spleen, stomach, and large intestine. The juice of fresh cucumber leaves can be used to heal burns, as can slices of cucumber placed gently against the affected part. Cucumber cools body heat. It is therefore useful for counteracting ailments due to heat in the lungs and stomach, such as acne, skin rashes, and dry, hot coughs.

Protein, 0.3 g; Fat, 0.1 g; Fiber, 0.3 g; Carbohydrate, 1.5 g; Vitamin A, 23 IU; Vitamin B_1, 0.02 mg; Vitamin B_2, 0.01 mg; Niacin, 0.2 mg; Vitamin C, 2 mg; Calcium, 7 mg; Phosphorus, 9 mg; Iron, 0.11 mg

Daikon (white radish)
Pungent and sweet (Metal and Earth), cool, weak Yang

Daikon affects the lungs and the stomach. It eliminates hot irritation of the throat and bronchi, and is therefore a useful remedy for coughs and laryngitis. It detoxifies and helps digestion, thus curing indigestion and diarrhea. Its juice also helps asthma patients.

Protein, 0.7 g; Fat, 0.1 g; Fiber, 0.8 g; Carbohydrate, 3.4 g; Vitamin A, 3 IU; Vitamin B_1, 0.06 mg; Vitamin B_2, 0.02 mg; Niacin, 0.5 mg; Vitamin C, 15 mg; Calcium, 35 mg; Phosphorus, 22 mg; Iron, 0.4 mg

Eggplant (aubergine)
Sweet (Earth), cool, balance of Yin and Yang

Eggplant nourishes the blood and qi and relieves pain, swelling, and heat. The raw juice is used as an application for softening and removing corns. In China eggplant is recommended for treating hemorrhages, ulcerations of the skin and gums, dysentery with blood, and anal bleeding.

Protein, 0.5 g; Fat, 0 g; Fiber, 0.6 g; Carbohydrate, 2.6 g; Vitamin A, 29 IU; Vitamin B_1, 0.04 mg; Vitamin B_2, 0.01 mg; Niacin, 0.2 mg; Vitamin C, 1 mg; Calcium, 15 mg; Phosphorus, 13 mg; Iron, 0.22 mg

Lettuce
Bitter and sweet (Fire and Earth), cool, Yin

Lettuce tones the blood and qi and dissipates heat. Because lettuce promotes the formation of body fluids, it is considered an effective diuretic and a remedy for poor lactation.

Protein, 0.2 g; Fat, 0 g; Fiber, 0.1 g; Carbohydrate, 0.4 g; Vitamin A, 146 IU; Vitamin B_1, 0.01 mg; Vitamin B_2, 0.01 mg; Niacin, 0 mg; Vitamin C, 1 mg; Calcium, –; Phosphorus, –; Iron, 0.04 mg

Onion, green (scallion)
Pungent and sweet (Metal and Earth), warm, strong Yang

Onion, a diaphoretic, affects the lungs and stomach. The white head of the scallion is used in many recipes for colds and nasal congestion. Although not as potent as garlic, onions are of the same family and exert the same therapeutic effects. In other words, they are antibiotics and blood thinners. Note that the younger and fresher the onion, the stronger its therapeutic properties.

Protein, 1.8 g; Fat, 0.1 g; Fiber, 0.6 g; Carbohydrate, 12.6 g; Vitamin A, 15 IU; Vitamin B_1, 0.08 mg; Vitamin B_2, 0.02 mg; Niacin, 0.5 mg; Vitamin C, 5 mg; Calcium, 40 mg; Phosphorus, 60 mg; Iron, 1.2 mg

Potato
Sweet (Earth), neutral, Yang

Potato nourishes the spleen, pancreas, blood, and qi. It soothes inflammation. Potato juice can be applied to burns both to cool and diminsh pain and facilitate healing.

Protein, 2.3 g; Fat, 0.1 g; Fiber, –; Carbohydrate, 20.1 g; Vitamin A, 0 IU; Vitamin B_1, 0.1 mg; Vitamin B_2, 0.04 mg; Niacin, 1.7 mg; Vitamin C, 22 mg; Calcium, 8 mg; Phosphorus, 52 mg; Iron, 0.85 mg

Pumpkin
Sweet (Earth), neutral, balance of Yin and Yang

Pumpkin is a mild diaphoretic. Because it is able to clear damp conditions, it is a good and often-used remedy for bronchial asthma. It is also taken to relieve abdominal pains during pregnancy.

Protein, 1.3 g; Fat, 0.3 g; Fiber, –; Carbohydrate, 9.9 g; Vitamin A, 26,908 IU; Vitamin B_1, 0.03 mg; Vitamin B_2, 0.07 mg; Niacin, 0.4 mg; Vitamin C, 5 mg; Calcium, 32 mg; Phosphorus, 42 mg; Iron, 1.7 mg

Shiitake mushroom
Sweet (Earth), neutral, weak Yang

Mushrooms have been an integral part of Chinese medicine for centuries. The earliest materia medica from over two thousand years ago describe the medicinal properties of more than twenty species. Hundreds more are treated in modern publications.[4] Among these, shiitake mushrooms, China's most common fungi, are mentioned as useful in treating vomiting, coughs, and urinary deficiencies. Regular consumption is also thought to prevent the development of cancer.

Because shiitake mushrooms are easily cultivated, they are used in everyday cooking as a tasty ingredient to enhance both meat and vegetarian dishes. Shiitake mushrooms are used in popular treatments for coughs, to prevent hardening of the arteries, as a diuretic, and to soothe irritation from food toxins.

Protein, 1.4 g; Fat, 0.2 g; Fiber, –; Carbohydrate, 11.3 g; Vitamin A, 0 IU; Vitamin B$_1$, 0.05 mg; Vitamin B$_2$, 0.19 mg; Niacin, 2.1 mg; Vitamin C, 1 mg; Calcium, 2 mg; Phosphorus, 44 mg; Iron, 0.26 mg

Spinach
Sweet (Earth), cool, balance of Yin and Yang

Spinach nourishes qi and the blood; its high iron content makes it a useful remedy for anemia. Spinach has a cool, glossy texture, which exerts a lubricating effect on ailments of a hot, dry nature, such as a dry and rasping cough, thirst, and red and dry mucus in the mouth and nose. Spinach also nourishes the intestines; this, coupled with its smooth texture, make it a good laxative.

Spinach broth is a remedy for intoxication. Spinach is often eaten to stop hair loss. Another of its recognized characteristics is that spinach arrests bleeding. It is therefore consumed as a remedy against nosebleed, as well as for anal bleeding.

Protein, 0.4 g; Fat, 0.1 g; Fiber, –; Carbohydrate, 0.7 g; Vitamin A, 1232 IU; Vitamin B$_1$, 0.01 mg; Vitamin B$_2$, 0.04 mg; Niacin, 0.1 mg; Vitamin C, 8 mg; Calcium, 16 mg; Phosphorus, 8 mg; Iron, 0.22 mg

Sweet potato
Sweet (Earth), neutral, Yang

Sweet potato nourishes the spleen, liver, blood, and qi. It is a valid remedy for constipation and for indigestion. Sweet potato soup will help to clear the head after drinking alcohol. Its diaphoretic effects render it effective against the common cold.

Protein, 2.7 g; Fat, 0.5 g; Fiber, –; Carbohydrate, 39.8 g; Vitamin A, 27,968 IU; Vitamin B$_1$, 0.09 mg; Vitamin B$_2$, 0.23 mg; Niacin, 1.1 mg; Vitamin C, 28 mg; Calcium, 35 mg; Phosphorus, 44 mg; Iron, 0.92 mg

Tomato
Sweet and sour (Earth and Wood), slightly cold, Yin

Tomato dissipates heat and stimulates the appetite and digestion. In China, raw tomato is served as an appetizer to promote digestion. It is prescribed to treat anemia, high blood pressure, constipation, and indigestion. A decoction made from the tomato plant is used to treat amoebic dysentery.

Protein, 1.1 g; Fat, 0.3 g; Fiber, 1.0 g; Carbohydrate, 5.3 g; Vitamin A, 1394 IU; Vitamin B$_1$, 0.07 mg; Vitamin B$_2$, 0.06 mg; Niacin, 0.7; Vitamin C, 22 mg; Calcium, 8 mg; Phosphorus, 29 mg; Iron, 0.59 mg

Water chestnut
Sweet (Earth), cold, Yin

Water chestnuts, a popular remedy for indigestion and hepatitis, also relieve fever. They are a useful source of nutrients for diabetics. Cut open and applied to the face, water chestnuts are used to cure acne. Eaten raw or drunk as juice, water chestnuts relieve sore throat and gums and canker sores.

Protein, 0.9 g; Fat, 0.1 g; Fiber, –; Carbohydrate, 14.8 g; Vitamin A, 0 IU; Vitamin B$_1$, 0.09 mg; Vitamin B$_2$, 0.12 mg; Niacin, 0.6 mg; Vitamin C, 3 mg; Calcium, 7 mg; Phosphorus, 39 mg; Iron, 0.37 mg

NUTS AND SEEDS

Nuts and seeds are storehouses of energy. They contain essential fatty acids and carbohydrates, and are rich in minerals and in vitamin E. Vitamin E is a powerful antioxidant that protects cells and nerves from aging and degeneration.

As with all foods, nuts and seeds are best eaten fresh. When freshly picked nuts are unavailable, it is best to select those that are still in their shells. Hulled and shelled nuts and seeds easily become rancid, thereby losing all nutrients and becoming difficult to digest. Nuts left in their shells can be consumed up to one year after harvesting.

Most nuts and seeds have warming properties. They are therefore particularly useful for treating cold-syndrome diseases and for fortifying the body in winter.

As with fruits and vegetables, it is best to eat organically grown nuts and seeds. Sprayed insecticides and poisons accumulate in seeds more readily than in the stem or fruit of plants.

Almonds
Bitter and sweet (Fire and Earth), warm, Yang

Almonds, common in northern China, are one of the foods richest in calcium and phosphorus. They nourish the blood and qi, and lubricate the lungs and bronchi.

Almonds and almond milk are commonly used to relieve coughs. According to tradition, almonds should be consumed to counteract the development of athlete's foot. Almond and chrysanthemum tea alleviates headaches.

Protein, 20.6 g; Fat, 52.10 g; Fiber, 4.58 g; Carbohydrate, 20.42 g; Vitamin A, 0 IU; Vitamin B$_1$, 0.21 mg; Vitamin B$_2$, 0.77 mg; Niacin, 3.52 mg; Vitamin C, traces; Calcium, 264 mg; Phosphorus, 520.96 mg; Iron, 3.66 mg

Caraway seeds
Slightly pungent (Metal), warm, Yang

Caraway seed stimulates the circulation of blood and qi. It affects the internal organs of digestion, in particular the stomach and kidneys.

Protein, 8 g; Fat, 6 g; Fiber, –; Carbohydrate, 22 g; Vitamin A, 160 IU; Vitamin B$_1$, 0.2 mg; Vitamin B$_2$, 0.2 mg; Niacin, 2 mg; Vitamin C, 0 mg; Calcium, 280 mg; Phosphorus, 240 mg; Iron, 6.8 mg

Chestnuts
Sweet (Earth), warm, Yang

Chestnuts fortify Yang and nourish qi and blood. Being warm, chestnuts dissipate cold-syndrome diseases. They are used as a remedy for diarrhea, especially when due to cold. They are also often used to treat nausea.

Protein, 4.22 g; Fat, 1.06 g; Fiber, 6 g; Carbohydrate, 48.93 g; Vitamin A, 200 IU; Vitamin B$_1$, 0.18 mg; Vitamin B$_2$, 0.18 mg; Niacin, 0.7 mg; Vitamin C, 35.2 mg; Calcium, 17.6 mg; Phosphorus, 95.04 mg; Iron, 1.41 mg

Peanuts
Sweet (Earth), neutral, Yang

Peanuts nourish qi and the blood. They strengthen and lubricate the lungs, and are often used to treat dry coughs. In China, peanuts are not normally served salted. Roasted or boiled peanuts stimulate the appetite, and for this reason are often served at the beginning of Chinese banquets as appetizers. Boiled peanuts with milk and honey is a common remedy both for stomachache and for gastritis. Peanut husks are used as a remedy for anemia.

Eaten fresh, peanuts alleviate coughs with catarrh. Peanuts are also recognized as a remedy for beriberi, and are often prescribed as part of a diet aimed at lowering blood pressure. Peanuts boiled with soymilk or eaten with pork are said to promote the secretion of milk after childbirth.

Protein, 25.7 g; Fat, 44.2 g; Fiber, 2.4 g; Carbohydrate, 23.6 g; Vitamin A, 0 IU; Vitamin B$_1$, 0.66 mg; Vitamin B$_2$, 0.14 mg; Niacin, 14.08 mg; Vitamin C, 0 mg; Calcium, 59.84 mg; Phosphorus, 383.68 mg; Iron, 3.24 mg

Sesame seeds
Sweet (Earth), neutral, balance of Yin and Yang

The sesame plant has been cultivated in China for five thousand years. The seeds are pressed to make sesame oil, prized all over China as the best oil for condiments and stir-frying. The seeds themselves are used extensively in traditional Chinese medicine. There are two varieties of sesame seeds: black and white. Although their functions are more or less the same, the black variety is usually preferred for medicinal purposes.

Sesame nourishes the blood and improves eyesight. It dispels evil wind, and dryness in the intestines. Sesame aids the production of body fluids and stimulates the secretion of maternal milk after childbirth. It reinforces the functions of the liver and helps to mainain black, shiny hair. Sesame is also used in remedies for general weakness, anemia, constipation, dizziness, ringing in the ears, hypertension, and chronic cough.

Protein, 16.8 g; Fat, 47.6 g; Fiber, –; Carbohydrate, 25.9 g; Vitamin A, 5 IU; Vitamin B$_1$, 1.19 mg; Vitamin B$_2$, 0.45 mg; Niacin, 5.25 mg; Vitamin C, 0 mg; Calcium, 129.5 mg; Phosphorus, 770 mg; Iron, 7.73 mg

Sunflower seeds
Sweet (Earth), neutral, mild Yang

Sunflower seeds regulate the action of the large intestine. They are useful in treating severe diarrhea and dysentery with blood in the stools. Sunflower seeds contain plenty of essential minerals, particularly zinc. One teapoon of crushed sunflower seeds dissolved in hot water and drunk as a tea will allow the skin pustules that erupt in measles and chicken pox to mature more rapidly. Two tablespoons of crushed sunflower seeds brewed in the same way is an effective laxative.

Protein, 22.88 g; Fat, 49.63 g; Fiber, –; Carbohydrate, 18.66 g; Vitamin A, 49.28 IU; Vitamin B$_1$, 2.29 mg; Vitamin B$_2$, 0.25 mg; Niacin, 4.58 mg; Vitamin C, –; Calcium, 116.16 mg; Phosphorus, 704 mg; Iron, 6.76 mg

Walnuts
Sweet (Earth), warm, Yang

Walnuts are a tonic for the blood and the kidneys. They lubricate the intestines and are thus a good remedy for constipation. Walnuts also alleviate asthma. They are often prescribed in China for male sexual problems such as seminal emission and impotence.

If chewed slowly, raw walnuts give some relief to a sore throat. Mixed with sesame seeds, ginger, and honey, they relieve stomach pains. A decoction of walnuts and fresh ginger is known to relieve fever and headache associated with the common cold.

Protein, 15 g; Fat, 56.67 g; Fiber, 2.1 g; Carbohydrate, 15.6 g; Vitamin A, 30 IU; Vitamin B$_1$, 0.48 mg; Vitamin B$_2$, 0.11 mg; Niacin, 0.7 mg; Vitamin C, 3 mg; Calcium, 83 mg; Phosphorus, 380 mg; Iron, 3.06 mg

GRAINS AND BEANS

Grains are at the base of the human food pyramid. Whole grains provide all our nutritional needs: proteins, carbohydrates, vitamins, enzymes, and minerals.

Being a major source of calories, every agriculture-based culture in the world has selected one of the grains as its preferred staple. In Europe the staple grain is wheat; in pre-Columbian America it was maize and amaranth; in India it is rice; in China it is rice in the south and wheat in the north.

Because whole, unhusked grains contain greater quantities of nutrients than polished or processed grains, it is preferable to consume all grains and cereals as close to their natural state as possible. One problem that may arise from eating whole grains is difficulty in digesting them. This may be partly overcome by thoroughly chewing grains. The process of digesting carbohydrates starts with the action of saliva in the mouth, which converts starch to more easily digestible maltose. The more time grains remain in the mouth, the greater the predigestive efficacy of saliva

Like nuts and seeds, beans are rich in carbohydrates, proteins, minerals, and enzymes. As with whole grains, beans are also difficult to digest and, once digested, are notorious for causing flatulence. Fortunately, several remedies exist. Thorough chewing is one of them. Another is to soak beans overnight before cooking, or until they sprout. Sprouting changes the beans' chemical composition. Although less energetic and cooler than unsprouted beans, they are easier to digest. A common antidote in China to their flatulence-causing properties is to eat beans with ginger; this prevents bloating. Another technique is not to add salt until cooking is almost complete—salt interferes with the proper cooking of the skin of most legumes, thereby rendering them tough and indigestible. One can also cook beans with fennel or cumin seed, which stimulate digestion and the metabolism.

Adzuki bean
Sour and sweet (Wood and Earth), neutral, balance of Yin and Yang

Adzuki beans are a classic remedy for beriberi. They are also used as a remedy for bloody stools, diarrhea, balancing hormones during menopause, aiding the secretion of milk after childbirth, and for athlete's foot.

Protein, 8.7 g; Fat, 0.1 g; Fiber, 0.5 g; Carbohydrate, 26 g; Vitamin A, 6 IU; Vitamin B_1, 0.13 mg; Vitamin B_2, 0.07 mg; Niacin, 0.8 mg; Vitamin C, 0 mg; Calcium, 182 mg; Phosphorus, 22 mg; Iron, 2.36 mg

Mung bean
Sweet (Earth), cool, balance of Yin and Yang

Mung beans dissipate heat, detoxify, and nourish the heart and stomach. They are a remedy for high blood pressure, hemorrhoids, headaches, and intoxication from alcohol, lead, or mild poisons. The recipe for detoxifying is to boil one-half to one pound of mung beans in water and take as a soup, with seasoning, or grind the same amount into a powder and mix with warm water.

Protein, 6.8 g; Fat, 0.5 g; Fiber, –; Carbohydrate, 10 g; Vitamin A, 28 IU; Vitamin B_1, 0.13 mg; Vitamin B_2, 0.07 mg; Niacin, 1.3 mg; Vitamin C, 1 mg; Calcium, 46 mg; Phosphorus, 140 mg; Iron, 1.62 mg

Rice
Sweet (Earth), neutral, weak Yang

Because rice is the staple dish in southern China, it would be quite surprising were it not recognized as having some therapeutic function within Chinese home remedies. Surprisingly, however, the therapeutic properties of rice turn out to be few. Polished rice is used as a base for various food remedies, usually as a sort of gruel or *congee*. On its own, rice can be eaten as a source of nourishing energy for the spleen and stomach, particularly when suffering from diarrhea and nausea. Two or three tablespoons of rice with a slice of fresh ginger, chewed slowly first thing in the morning on an empty stomach, can help allay morning sickness.

Unfortunately, the relatively recent use of chemical weed killers in the rice-growing industry suggests that commercially grown rice may be harmful to one's health. Rice is grown in rich, fertile soil in a few inches of water, ideal conditions for weeds and other parasites. Until a few years ago these weeds were removed by hand by cohorts of women workers who systematically damaged their bodies by wading, bent double, through the rice paddies, pulling at the weeds—necessary work that no one wanted to do. Chemical weed killers eliminated the need for any further human intervention. Yet the use of these weed killers translates as health risks to the consumer. In order to work, weed killers must be added to the rice crop in such concentrations that the amount of poison present in every grain of unhusked rice is twenty times the danger level for human consumption.[5]

Most of the weed-killing poison settles in the husk. If you eat polished rice, you eliminate the poisons as well as the vitamins.

Polished rice: Protein, 6.8 g; Fat, 0.5 g; Fiber, 0.2 g; Carbohydrate, 78.2 g; Vitamin A, 0 IU; Vitamin B_1, 0.06 mg; Vitamin B_2, 0.06 mg; Niacin, 1.9 mg; Vitamin C, 0 mg; Calcium, 10 mg; Phosphorus, 160 mg; Iron, 3.1 mg

Unpolished rice: Protein, 7.5 g; Fat, 1.0 g; Fiber, 0.6 g; Carbohydrate, 76.7 g; Vitamin A, 2 IU; Vitamin B_1, 0.21 mg; Vitamin B_2, 0.16 mg; Niacin, 1.9 g; Vitamin C, 0 mg; Calcium, 10 mg; Phosphorus, 190 mg; Iron, 3.2 mg

Rice bran
Pungent (Metal), warm,
strong Yang

Rice bran, a diaphoretic, dissipates cold and affects the stomach and intestines. An ancient remedy for beriberi, rice bran is commonly used in China for treating constipation. When mixed with honey, it provides relief from coughs.

Protein, 11.9 g; Fat, 21.7 g; Fiber, –; Carbohydrate, 45.6 g; Vitamin A, 0 IU; Vitamin B_1, 2.21 mg; Vitamin B_2, 0.26 mg; Niacin, 31.2 mg; Vitamin C, 0 mg; Calcium, 355 mg; Phosphorus, –; Iron, 7.88 mg

Soybean
Sweet (Earth), neutral, weak Yang

Soybeans have been used medicinally in China for five thousand years. Because of their high protein content and ease of digestion, they are one of the most valuable ingredients in Chinese cuisine. Soybeans energize the entire body, nourishing the spleen and lubricating the intestines. They build muscles and regulate body fat, and are therefore valuable for low-fat and weight-reducing diets.

Soybeans are commonly used as a remedy for malnutrition, poor digestion, diarrhea, and high cholesterol. A product of soybeans used extensively in Chinese cuisine and medicine is tofu.

Protein, 11 g; Fat, 5.8 g; Fiber, –; Carbohydrate, 10 g; Vitamin A, 140 IU; Vitamin B_1, 0.23 mg; Vitamin B_2, 0.14 mg; Niacin, 1.1 mg; Vitamin C, 15 mg; Calcium, 131 mg; Phosphorus, 142 mg; Iron, 2.25 mg

Tofu

Sweet (Earth), cool, balance of
Yin and Yang

Tofu (pronounced **doe**-fu in China) is made from dried, crushed soybeans that are boiled and then coagulated to form solid tofu and soymilk. Tofu is soft and pudding-like; the rubbery skin that forms on the surface during coagulation, called bamboo *tofu*, is an important ingredient of Chinese vegetarian cuisine.

Tofu dissipates heat and dryness. It tones the entire body and is particularly nourishing to the blood and qi. Tofu is used to treat chronic amoebic dysentery; anemia; stubborn, dry cough; nausea; vomiting; intoxication; high blood pressure; insufficient lactation; and arthritis and rheumatism. According to recent Western research, soy protein's ability to clear cholesterol from the blood is unsurpassed by any other foodstuff.[6]

Protein, 11 g; Fat, 2.3 g; Fiber, –; Carbohydrate, 11 g; Vitamin A, 209 IU; Vitamin B$_1$, 0.2 mg; Vitamin B$_2$, 0.13 mg; Niacin, 0.5 mg; Vitamin C, 0 mg; Calcium, 258 mg; Phosphorus, 239 mg; Iron, 13.9 mg

---

MEAT AND POULTRY

Chinese people consume little meat, although tourists to China often come away with a very different impression. Tourist meals are about 50 percent meat. The reason for this is simple: Chinese hospitality.

Chinese people are aware of Westerners' partiality to meat and will thus provide plenty of it to "foreign friends." We ourselves eat meat perhaps once a week; when we do it is with therapeutic or nutritional intent. The life of animals is respected both by Buddhists and Taoists. Furthermore, animal qi is considered by some to be bad for humans, and for that reason rituals exist for the slaying of animals. Because misfortune is said to come to one who kills an animal, only old people whose life force is ebbing anyway are supposed to practice butchery. Young people should not even be present when an animal is killed. If a young person must kill an animal, he must bite hard on the blade of the killing knife before using it on the beast. A disculpatory jingle is recited to the animal before it is killed: *"Bu yuan ni, bu yuan wo, guan yuan ni zhu jia mai gei wo."* No blame on you, no blame on me, just blame your master for selling you to me." Afterward the blood is collected, steamed, and eaten by the butcher as an act of penitence.

Another taboo is that one should never eat an animal that has not been killed after the first attempt. If the first cut missed or only injured the animal, it is said to mean that the gods are protecting it, and it should, if still possible, be allowed to live. If the injury is too great, it should be killed with a second stroke but not eaten.

Beef

Sweet (Earth), neutral, Yang

Considered to be of the Earth element, beef builds the qi and blood, tones yin, and strengthens muscles. Beef is prescribed as a general tonic for weakness and convalescence. It is a specific treatment for lumbago, chronic diarrhea, anorexia, and low blood pressure.

Until recently, beef was rarely eaten in China. Indeed, few people know that the taboos that exist in India about the consumption of cow flesh also applied in China before the thirteenth century; beef became more popular only after the Mongolian conquest of China in A.D. 1215.[7]

The Mongolian grasslands were ideal for cattle and sheep grazing; the Mongolians have therefore always been meat eaters. They brought their meat-eating habits with them to China, thus influencing local cuisine and doing away with the old taboos forever. Today beef is consumed without any qualms in China, with the exception of those relating to expense.

Protein, 25 g; Fat, 27 g; Fiber, 0 g; Carbohydrate, 0 g; Vitamin A, 0 IU; Vitamin B$_1$, 0.05 mg; Vitamin B$_2$, 0.2 mg; Niacin, 4.1 mg; Vitamin C, 0 mg; Calcium, 11 mg; Phosphorus, 170 mg; Iron, 3.1 mg

Chicken
Sweet (Earth), warm, Yang

Chicken assists circulation of blood and qi. It is used in cures for diarrhea and dysentery. Chicken is also prescribed for problems as varied as anorexia; diabetes; leukorrhea; slow lactation; weakness; and liver, kidney, and urinary deficiencies.

Protein, 20 g; Fat, 2.7 g; Fiber, 0 g; Carbohydrate, 0 g; Vitamin A, 0 IU; Vitamin B$_1$, 0.1 mg; Vitamin B$_2$, 0.24 mg; Niacin, 5.6 mg; Vitamin C, 0 mg; Calcium, 15 mg; Phosphorus, 188 mg; Iron, 1.8 mg

Pork
Sweet and salty (Earth and Water), neutral, mild Yang

So common is the pig to rural family life that the Chinese character for family depicts a pig under a roof. Pork is the most common meat consumed in China. Consequently, it figures prominently in popular food remedies as well.

Pork is used for constipation, debility, malnutrition and emaciation, dry cough, and diabetes. It is also prescribed for combating hyperacidity and gastritis, male sexual problems, and overly dry skin.

Protein, 22.3 g; Fat, 26.1 g; Fiber, 0 g; Carbohydrate, 0 g; Vitamin A, 8 IU; Vitamin B$_1$, 0.52 mg; Vitamin B$_2$, 0.3 mg; Niacin, 3.9 mg; Vitamin C, 0 mg; Calcium, 8 mg; Phosphorus, 206 mg; Iron, 1.19 mg

Mutton
Sweet (Earth), warm, Yang

Mutton nourishes qi and the blood. It is considered a good tonic for conditions of general weakness and fatigue. Mutton is the preferred meat for curing male sexual weaknesses such as frequent nocturnal emission and premature ejaculation. It is also prescribed for indigestion, pains in the abdomen, and all cold-syndrome ailments.

Protein, 21.5 g; Fat, 16.1 g; Fiber, 0 g; Carbohydrate, 0 g; Vitamin A, –; Vitamin B$_1$, 0.13 mg; Vitamin B$_2$, 2.3 mg; Niacin, 4.7 mg; Vitamin C, 0 mg; Calcium, 9 mg; Phosphorus, 177 mg; Iron, 1.4 mg

FISH

In China, fish is considered to be one of the most wholesome foods. Fish is also considered to be a symbol of wealth and abundance; the word for fish (yu) is pronounced just like the word meaning "abundance." The golden carp, or goldfish (yu jing), is particularly auspicious because the word sounds similar to the words meaning "abundant gold"—hence the great number of goldfish images one sees on the walls of many Chinese restaurants around the world. Fish are also a positive symbol in Buddhist iconography. For Buddhists they represent freedom from the chains of the material world.

The most commonly eaten fish in China is carp; they are plentiful, as they breed with ease in ponds and rice paddies. Shrimp are among the most prized fish, however, so accorded for their strong Yang energy. Other popular fish are eel, clams, crab, and abalone. The last, however, is not commonly found outside China. Abalone is difficult to digest and does not feature in any of our remedies. We shall not, therefore, describe it here.

Carp
Sweet (Earth), cold, Yang

Carp meat nourishes the blood and qi and affects the stomach, kidneys, and spleen. It is a diuretic. Carp also promotes lactation after childbirth.

Protein, 17.75 g; Fat, 5.6 g; Fiber, –; Carbohydrate, 0 g; Vitamin A, 8 IU; Vitamin B_1, –; Vitamin B_2, –; Niacin, –; Vitamin C, 1 mg; Calcium, 41 mg; Phosphorus, 410 mg; Iron, 1.23 mg

Clam
Salty (Water), cold, Yin

Clam meat dissipates toxic heat and dryness. A light, cooling meat, it promotes the flow and distribution of body fluids, thus acting as a detoxifier. Clam meat exerts a beneficial effect on the stomach, lowers high blood pressure, and is known to resolve vaginal bleeding and discharge (leukorrhea). It is sometimes prescribed for treating hemorrhoids.

Protein, 12.8 g; Fat, 1.4 g; Fiber, 0 g; Carbohydrate, 3.4 g; Vitamin A, 110 IU; Vitamin B_1, 0.1 mg; Vitamin B_2, 0.18 mg; Niacin, 1.6 mg; Vitamin C, 0 mg; Calcium, 96 mg; Phosphorus, 139 mg; Iron, 7 mg

Crab
Salty (Water), cold, Yin

Crab is a cold meat and is therefore nearly always cooked with ginger, which is warming, for balance. However, if you are suffering from a toxic heat syndrome, crab has the effect of dissipating the heat. It relieves heat rashes and pustules on the skin.

Protein, 16.9 g; Fat, 2.9 g; Fiber, 0 g; Carbohydrate, 1.3 g; Vitamin A, 0 IU; Vitamin B_1, 0.05 mg; Vitamin B_2, 0.06 mg; Niacin, 2.5 mg; Vitamin C, 0 mg; Calcium, 45 mg; Phosphorus, 182 mg; Iron, 0.9 mg

Eel
Sweet (Earth), warm, Yang

Eel is considered to be a good tonic for the body and qi, and is thus often taken for fatigue or debilitation. It is also prescribed for rheumatic disorders.

Protein, 18.3 g; Fat, 11.5 g; Fiber, –; Carbohydrate, 0 g; Vitamin A, 1034 IU; Vitamin B_1, 0.15 mg; Vitamin B_2, 0.04 mg; Niacin, 3.5 mg; Vitamin C, 6 mg; Calcium, 19.8 mg; Phosphorus, 213 mg; Iron, 0.5 mg

Shrimp
Sweet (Earth), warm, Yang

Shrimp meat dissipates cold, tones Yang, and removes stagnation in the flow of qi. In China, shrimp is valued first and foremost for enhancing male sexual energy, and thus correcting impotence. Because of its strong Yang energy however, it will make seminal emission and premature ejaculation worse. The strong energy of shrimp is an aid during convalescence.

Protein, 20.2 g; Fat, 1.75 g; Fiber, –; Carbohydrate, 0.9 g; Vitamin A, –; Vitamin B_1, 0.02 mg; Vitamin B_2, 0.03 mg; Niacin, 2.6 mg; Vitamin C, –; Calcium, 51 mg; Phosphorus, 204 mg; Iron, 2.39 mg

EGG

Eggs are birds in the making. As such, they are extremely high-protein foods with powerful nutritional and therapeutic effects.

Eggs are made of three different constituents: the yolk, the white, and the shell. The latter is usually discarded by cooks in the West. In China, however, eggshell has a variety of uses. Eggshell ground into a fine powder and taken with meals decreases gastric acid, and is thus a remedy for gastric and duodenal ulcers. Ground eggshell dissolved in *jiu* (Chinese rice wine, or Japanese *sake*) cures stomach problems. Sterilized ground eggshell applied to a wound will arrest bleeding.

Because milk is not commonly drunk in China, eggshell is often used as a remedy for rickets—insufficient vitamin D leading to defective bone growth—and calcium deficiency in children.

Whole egg
Sweet (Earth), neutral, Yin

Considered to be a highly nutritious and energetic food, egg dissipates dryness and nourishes the blood and qi. It is used in a wide variety of remedies, from asthma to coughs and the common cold. It is also included in remedies for dysentery, diarrhea, constipation, hepatitis, anemia, nausea and vomiting, and insomnia.

Protein, 6.1 g; Fat, 5.5 g; Fiber, 0 g; Carbohydrate, 0.6 g; Vitamin A, 260 IU; Vitamin B$_1$, 0.04 mg; Vitamin B$_2$, 0.14 mg; Niacin, 0 mg; Vitamin C, 0 mg; Calcium, 28 mg; Phosphorus, 90 mg; Iron, 1.04 mg

Egg white
Sweet (Earth), cool, weak Yin

Egg white has a cooling effect; it also moistens and soothes excessive dryness of the eyes, throat, and lungs. By cooling and moisturizing, egg white effectively detoxifies the entire body. It is also considered to be a good remedy for anemia.

One egg white drunk raw every morning keeps constipation at bay. Mix it with fruit juice if you find the white distasteful on its own. In China, raw egg white mixed with rice wine is an application for scalds and burns.

Protein, 3.4 g; Fat, 0 g; Fiber, 0 g; Carbohydrate, 0.4 g; Vitamin A, 0 IU; Vitamin B$_1$, 0 mg; Vitamin B$_2$, 0.09 mg; Niacin, 0 mg; Vitamin C, 0 mg; Calcium, 4 mg; Phosphorus, 4 mg; Iron, 0.01 mg

Egg yolk
Sweet (Earth), neutral, medium Yang

Egg yolks are considered nourishing for the liver, heart, and kidneys. They are more effective than a whole egg for curing vomiting and diarrhea—one remedy for continual vomiting is to swallow half a dozen raw or underboiled egg yolks in a single sitting.

Protein, 2.8 g; Fat, 5.6 g; Fiber, 0 g; Carbohydrate, 0 g; Vitamin A, 313 IU; Vitamin B$_1$, 0.4 mg; Vitamin B$_2$, 0.07 mg; Niacin, 0 mg; Vitamin C, 0 mg; Calcium, 26 mg; Phosphorus, 86 mg; Iron, 0.9 mg

HERBS AND SPICES

All cultures use herbs and spices in their cuisine. China is no exception. Some, such as ginger, cilantro, and garlic, have been used since antiquity. Others, like red or cayenne pepper, made their way to China after their discovery on the American continent, and have been used with great success ever since.

Herbs and spices serve two main purposes. They add or enhance flavor and they exert specific therapeutic effects. These effects are different for every herb and spice. Cinnamon and pepper, for example, are Yang and hot, peppermint and marjoram are Yin and cool.

Basil
Pungent (Metal), warm, ascending Yang

Basil promotes circulation of qi and blood, helps digestion, and reinforces the lungs, spleen, and stomach. Basil is not common in China. It is, however, known to traditional medicine, and is sometimes used as a treatment for abdominal pains, bloating, and diarrhea.

Protein, 0 g; Fat, 4 g; Fiber, 0 g; Carbohydrate, 2 g; Vitamin A, 80 IU; Vitamin B$_1$, 0 mg; Vitamin B$_2$, 0.2 mg; Niacin, 0 mg; Vitamin C, 20 mg; Calcium, 140 mg; Phosphorus, 10 mg; Iron, 11.8 mg

Cilantro (coriander or Chinese parsley)
Pungent (Metal), warm, Yang

Cilantro is used as a seasoning in many dishes, and particularly with seafood. Besides enhancing the flavor, cilantro serves to balance the cold effect of clams and crab. Cilantro's strong smell and flavor makes it a valuable breath freshener. It is also used in China to quicken the rash in measles: you can either wash the patient with a warm cilantro brew or use it liberally when preparing the patient's food.

Protein, 0.16 g; Fat, 0 g; Fiber, –; Carbohydrate, 0.16 g; Vitamin A, 185 IU; Vitamin B$_1$, 0 mg; Vitamin B$_2$, 0.02 mg; Niacin, 0 mg; Vitamin C, 0 mg; Calcium, 6.7 mg; Phosphorus, 1.6 mg; Iron, 0.13 mg

Cinnamon
Sweet and pungent (Earth and Metal), hot, Yang

Cinnamon nourishes the spleen, kidneys, and bladder.

Protein, 2 g; Fat, 2 g; Fiber, –; Carbohydrate, 36 g; Vitamin A, 120 IU; Vitamin B$_1$, 0 mg; Vitamin B$_2$, 0 mg; Niacin, 0 mg; Vitamin C, 20 mg; Calcium, 560 mg; Phosphorus, 20 mg; Iron, 17.6 mg

Clove
Pungent (Metal), warm, Yang that pushes downward

Clove affects the internal organs of digestion, the stomach and kidneys in particular. It is a warming spice that relieves hiccups, nausea, and stomach problems.

Protein, 2 g; Fat, 8 g; Fiber, –; Carbohydrate, 26 g; Vitamin A, 220 IU; Vitamin B$_1$, 0 mg; Vitamin B$_2$, 0.2 mg; Niacin, 0 mg; Vitamin C, 40 mg; Calcium, 280 mg; Phosphorus, 40 mg; Iron, 3.6 mg

Dill seed
Pungent (Metal), warm, Yang

Dill seed tones and regulates qi. A diaphoretic, it is particularly useful for warming the spleen and kidneys. Dill seed is used to treat vomiting, hiccups, and anorexia. Its warming effect counteracts abdominal and stomach pains due to cold.

Protein, 6 g; Fat, 6 g; Fiber, 0 g; Carbohydrate, 24 g; Vitamin A, 20 IU; Vitamin B$_1$, 0.2 mg; Vitamin B$_2$, 0.2 mg; Niacin, 0.2 mg; Vitamin C, 0 mg; Calcium, 640 mg; Phosphorus, 120 mg; Iron, 100 mg

Garlic
Pungent (Metal), warm, strong Yang

Garlic, a diaphoretic, warms the lungs, stomach, and spleen and promotes circulation of qi. The antibiotic effects of garlic have been recognized worldwide since antiquity.[8] Northern Chinese chew several cloves of raw garlic with their meals whenever they suspect poor sanitary conditions. If obliged to drink contaminated water, they chew a clove or two of garlic first, swallowing the juice and spitting out the fiber.

Because it destroys worms and bacteria, garlic is used as a remedy for diarrhea and chronic amoebic dysentery. Garlic is also an anticoagulant; taken daily, a clove or two of garlic can guard against blood clots, and thus can prevent heart attack or thrombosis. Garlic lowers cholesterol. As a sweat inducer (diaphoretic), garlic is frequently included in recipes for the common cold and influenza. Recent evidence suggests that garlic may also boost the immune system and slow the growth of tumors.[9]

For best effects, eat garlic raw. Many (though not all) of its benefits are lost through cooking. To counteract the unpleasant odor of garlic on the breath, most Chinese people will recommend chewing green tea leaves. Fresh dates or persimmon are said to banish the smell. You may also rinse the mouth with vinegar or drink a glass of milk to counteract the strong odor.

Protein, 6.3 g; Fat, 0.1 g; Fiber, 0.8 g; Carbohydrate, 29.8 g; Vitamin A, 0 IU; Vitamin B$_1$, 0.06 mg; Vitamin B$_2$, 0.23 mg; Niacin, 0.4 mg; Vitamin C, 13 mg; Calcium, 30 mg; Phosphorus, 310 mg; Iron, 1.3 mg

Ginger
Pungent (Metal), warm (dry ginger: hot), strong outward-moving Yang

Ginger acts on the lungs, stomach, and spleen. It disperses cold and relieves nausea; a slice of ginger or some ginger juice taken before a boat, car, or plane trip suppresses motion sickness. Ginger aids digestion; a slice or two chewed after a heavy meal combats indigestion and flatulence. Ginger is a powerful diaphoretic and a strong anticoagulant; a few slices of ginger taken daily can guard against blood clots, thus preventing heart attack or thrombosis. As a sweat inducer (diaphoretic), ginger is a

useful remedy for the common cold and influenza.

Note that fresh ginger contains volatile oils not present in the dried variety.

Protein, 2.3 g; Fat, 0.9 g; Fiber, 2.4 g; Carbohydrate, 12.3 g; Vitamin A, 40 IU; Vitamin B$_1$, 0.06 mg; Vitamin B$_2$, 0.03 mg; Niacin, 0.6 mg; Vitamin C, 0 mg; Calcium, 20 mg; Phosphorus, 60 mg; Iron, 2.6 mg

Ginseng
Sweet and slightly bitter (Earth and Fire), warm, weak Yang

The word *ginseng* is an anglicized pronunciation of the Chinese words *ren sheng*, meaning "root (or spirit) of man." Indeed, since ancient times in China ginseng has been used for building up the human spirit. Ginseng stimulates the nervous system, improving mental concentration, stamina, and memory. It builds resistance to disease and treats a variety of conditions ranging from colds to heart disease.

There exist two varieties of ginseng. *Panax ginseng*, a native of Asia, has been used in China for centuries. The other, *Panax quinquefolius*, is native to North America, where it has been cultivated since 1870.[10] Although Asian ginseng is recognized as the stronger of the two, in China American ginseng is frequently favored over the Asian variety. This is not because of some common human trait to regard things that come from overseas as better than that which is homegrown. Unless you are seriously ill or completely depleted of energy, Asian ginseng is too powerful. The American variety gives a steadier and less overpowering energy boost.

Ginseng may be taken in soups or with vegetable dishes. It can be brewed as a tea or macerated in a bottle of rice wine and sipped as a tonic. Dry ginseng is taken to treat morning sickness. Ginseng tea excites the heart and brain and stimulates the appetite. Eating ginseng improves sexual functions in both men and women—indeed, there are only a few conditions for which ginseng is not useful. Ginseng is a stimulant and an antidiuretic. It should therefore **not** be taken for kidney problems, insomnia, high blood pressure, and fever.

Protein, 6.5 g; Fat, 0.3 g; Fiber, –; Carbohydrate, 6 g; Vitamin A, 0 IU; Vitamin B$_1$, 0.02 mg; Vitamin B$_2$, 0.02 mg; Niacin, 0.3 mg; Vitamin C, 1.7 mg; Calcium, 7 mg; Phosphorus, 11.6 mg; Iron, 0.2 mg

Licorice
Sweet (Earth), neutral, Yang

Licorice, one of the most important ingredients in traditional Chinese herbal medicine, acts as a catalyst and regulates the effects of other herbal remedies. Its soothing characteristics are known to counteract toxins, and to have a calming effect on a body wracked by acute symptoms of a disease. Licorice invigorates the functions of the heart and lungs; it lubricates the lungs, soothing chronic and irritable coughs, and aids digestion by protecting the spleen and the lining of the stomach.

Licorice is frequently used as an antiphlogisitic (anti-inflammatory) for sore throat, boils, and irritation of the skin. It can also be useful as an antidote to poisoning by too many medicines or herbal drugs.

Licorice is not a common ingredient in American cuisine. Nutrient values for licorice are therefore not available.

Peppermint
Pungent (Metal), cool, Yang

Peppermint rises and affects the upper body, particularly the lungs. It also exerts a purifying effect on the organs of digestion and on the liver. It is an aid to digestion and

an efficient painkiller. Drink peppermint tea to cool you down in summer; the leaves may be chewed both to freshen the breath and to relieve toothache and mouth sores. Rub a little peppermint oil or fresh juice on your forehead and temples to relieve headache; drop a few drops in your ear for earache; rub some on mosquito bites to relieve itching.

Peppermint is not a common enough ingredient in American culinary practice to find nutrient value statistics.

SWEETENERS

Nearly everybody in America believes that sugar is bad for you. In China, however, sugar is frequently used as a lubricant or as a key ingredient in many food cures. The reason for this difference is that, in the United States, sugar is found in bread, soft drinks, and canned foods, and is often added indiscriminately to savory food preparations. It is thus consumed in vast quantities. Large quantities of sugar are deleterious to health.

Small quantities of sugar, on the other hand, exert a beneficial effect. Sugar soothes the stomach and spleen. It strengthens the qi and blood, and provides energy to the body.

Brown sugar
Sweet (Earth), warm, medium Yang

Useful as an energizing tonic, brown sugar nourishes qi and promotes circulation of both qi and blood. It nourishes the liver, spleen, and stomach. Mixed with rice wine, brown sugar raises low blood pressure.

Genuine brown sugar is less damaging than white sugar (sucrose) because some of the minerals from the original sugar cane are intact. The less refined the sugar you consume, the better. Undoubtedly the best sugar source is blackstrap molasses, the syrup left over after the sucrose (white sugar) has been extracted. Molasses contains all the nutrients and minerals of sugar cane in a more concentrated form. Sugar products are rare in China, however, and molasses is virtually unknown. It does not therefore appear in any Chinese home remedy.

It should also be noted that what is often sold commercially as brown sugar is merely the white refined variety, with some molasses added for coloring.

Protein, 0.1 g; Fat, 0.2 g; Fiber, 0 g; Carbohydrate, 9.1 g; Vitamin A, 6 IU; Vitamin B$_1$, 0 mg; Vitamin B$_2$, 0.002 mg; Niacin, 0 mg; Vitamin C, 0 mg; Calcium, 10 mg; Phosphorus, 10 mg; Iron, 1.1 mg. Note that these figures vary according to the degree of refinement.

White sugar
Sweet (Earth), neutral, medium Yang

Sugar's dual function in Chinese remedies is to sweeten otherwise unpalatable dishes and to give a quick rush of energy. It is said to lubricate the lungs, produce fluids, and nourish the spleen and liver. Sugar syrup (ordinary sugar boiled in water) is used in China to treat stomachache.

It should be noted that, in the Chinese diet, sugar is consumed in much smaller quantities than in the average American diet. Even though it appears as a main ingredient in several home remedies, it is best to refrain from taking any additional white sugar. We consume so much of it in the form of soft drinks, sweets, and industrially prepared foods that we still take far more than is good for us.

These are some of the drawbacks of eating white sugar. White sugar needs vitamins of the B complex in order to metabolize, so its consumption depletes your B vitamins. As well, the proper digestion of sugar is dependent upon calcium. White sugar can therefore deplete your bone calcium, including the calcium of your teeth. Sugar also causes dental damage because it forms a plaque on the teeth, which produces an acid that corrodes the teeth. Sugar raises cholesterol and triglycerides, which can be dangerous for the heart. Sugar increases uric acid in the bloodstream, a precursor to gout. Sugar combined with a salty diet raises blood pressure. Too much refined sugar overworks the pancreas, leading to its exhaustion and the possibility of diabetes.

Because sugar contains no vitamins in and of itself, and in fact depletes the body's nutrients in the process of metabolizing, it is best not to indulge in white sugar too often.

BEVERAGES

The most common beverage in China is tea, green tea being the most popular. Water is drunk, of course, but not icy cold. Indeed, it is usually sipped steaming hot, or at least warm. In China it is believed that cold water blocks digestion, whereas hot water aids circulation and dissolves fats.

Alcoholic beverages are consumed without qualms, often for social reasons but frequently for purely therapeutic purposes. The most common form of alcohol is distilled rice wine. Beer is also very popular. Grape wine is produced in China in small quantities, but has not yet made its way onto the Chinese dinner table.

Milk
Sweet (Earth), neutral, mild Yang

Chinese people do not drink much milk. This fact may account for the low levels of calcium among Chinese children, and the subsequent problem of weak bones. During our research we came across a number of remedies for this deficiency, from bone gruel to mashed eggshells. We have not included these simply because we do not believe that weak bones due to lack of calcium is a problem in the United States, where milk and milk products are consumed in abundance. Also, in only two of the counties surveyed were dairy products consumed in significant quantities, those being Tuoli in the predominantly Muslim and Ugyur region of northwest China and Xianghuang Qi in inner Mongolia. Neither is within the historical boundaries of China. Residents of Tuoli obtain 52.6 percent of their calories and 72.5 percent of their protein from milk and dairy products.

As a matter of interest, unless one is allergic to milk products or is lactose-intolerant, large consumption of dairy products appears to have no detrimental effects on health. The positive effects, on the other hand, are many.

Milk acts as a tonic for the stomach and lungs. It lubricates the intestines and thus counteracts constipation. It is easy to digest and facilitates digestion in general. It has a mild, sedative effect and is thus a remedy for insomnia.

Protein, 3.5 g; Fat, 3.9 g (whole), 0.1 g (nonfat); Fiber, 0 g; Carbohydrate, 4.9 g; Vitamin A, 160 IU; Vitamin B$_1$, 0.04 mg; Vitamin B$_2$, 0.17 mg; Niacin, 0.1 mg; Vitamin C, 1 mg; Calcium, 118 mg; Phosphorus, 93 mg; Iron, 0.1 mg

Tea, green and black
Bitter and sweet (Fire and Earth), cold, Yin

Tea originated in China in ancient times—its botanical name, *Camellia sinensis* (Chinese camellia) tells us as much. Tea was probably first used as a flavoring for the unpleasant tasting water of the Yelow River basin.[11] It was soon discovered that, as well as rendering water drinkable, tea was a nervous system stimulant and an aid to digestion. It has been much prized both as a drink and as a health aid ever since.[12]

All tea, green and black, comes from the same plant; the differences between varieties depends on two main factors. The first of these is habitat conditions, including the soil and climate. The second factor is the degree of processing that the tea leaves undergo between plucking and packaging. Green teas are the least processed: the leaves are "withered" (naturally dried) and then packaged. Oolong teas are withered and then slightly fermented. Lapsang souchong tea is withered, fermented, and smoked. Black teas are withered, fermented, and dried.

Tea is recognized as a diuretic and a mild stimulant. In 1991, studies in cancer research carried out by Dr. Alan Conney demonstrated that tea may also help in combating cancer. Three groups of mice were administered high doses of cancer-inducing drugs with their food. One group of mice was given nothing but water to drink. Another drank black, fermented tea, and a third group drank only green tea. At the end of the sixteen-week experiment all the mice were dissected and examined for cancerous tumors. While the water-drinking and black-tea-drinking mice each had, on average, eighty-five tumors in their bodies, the green-tea-drinking group had developed only fifteen tumorous growths, 80 percent less than the others.

In a second experiment Dr. Conney exposed the mice to strong ultraviolet rays. Ninety percent of the water-drinking mice developed skin cancer, while less than 30 percent of the tea drinkers were affected by the disease. Studies conducted in Israel,

Norway, and Japan have indicated that tea might also be beneficial in bringing down cholesterol levels.

Tea is used in China to cure headaches, colds, indigestion, dysentery, and acute gastroenteritis. Ground into a powder and applied externally to the skin two or three times a day, tea leaves are said to eliminate herpes zoster. On the downside, tea can cause constipation. Note that green tea, untreated and unfermented, is said to be better than black, smoked, or flavored teas.

The following nutritional values are for black tea only. Green tea is just now making a wider presence in the American market. As a consequence, nutritional values for green tea are not shown in any of the reference books currently available. Although no precise figures are given here, green tea is known to contain thiamine, riboflavin, niacin, folic acid and biotin, potassium, manganese, magnesium, copper, zinc, and sodium.

Protein, 0 g; Fat, 0 g; Fiber, 0 g; Carbohydrate, 0 g; Vitamin A, 0 IU; Vitamin B_1, 0 mg; Vitamin B_2, 0.03 mg; Niacin, 0 mg; Vitamin C, 6 mg; Calcium, 0 mg; Phosphorus, 1 mg; Iron, 0.04 mg

Wine

Sweet, bitter, and pungent (Earth, Fire, and Metal), warm, Yang

The term *wine* here refers not to grape wine but to spirit—generally rice spirit or that of sorghum or other grain.

Wine may be taken alone in order to stimulate blood circulation, relieve cold-syndrome diarrhea, or alleviate arthritic problems. It influences the heart and the liver, and, to a lesser extent, the stomach and the lungs. However, since ancient times medicinal herbs, roots, and other

ingredients have been macerated in wine in order to treat specific ailments. In China it is believed that any ingredient that you can prepare with a rice congee or gruel can also be macerated in wine. The congee will affect qi, while the wine will affect blood circulation.

Wine used for medical purposes should be between 50°f and 60°f. It is normally white, however, on occasion yellow wine is used. Wine has no nutritive value.

CONDIMENTS

Condiments are used the world over for the sole purpose of enhancing the flavors of foods. A flavor enhancer frequently associated with Chinese cuisine is monosodium glutamate (MSG)—the allergic reaction associated with an overconsumption of MSG is often referred to as "Chinese restaurant syndrome." In actual fact, in China only poor cooks add MSG to food in order to improve their otherwise uninteresting preparations. MSG has no flavor of its own, but exerts its effect directly on human taste buds so that we experience meats, fish, and vegetable dishes as more savory.

In spite of extensive negative press in recent years, MSG has no adverse effects unless you happen to be allergic to it, suffer from arteriosclerosis or high blood pressure, or consume it in massive quantities.* However, although MSG may not be as bad for us as many people believe, it serves no useful health purpose either. It therefore has no place in any of the recipes described in this volume except one: Chinese chicken

*It is the sodium that one needs to avoid in the case of arteriosclerosis and high blood pressure.

salad (see page 193). This hot mustard-based dish is assured an extra kick with the addition of a few grains of MSG.

Many other condiments serve important therapeutic purposes.

Olive
Sweet and sour (Earth and Wood),
neutral, balance of Yin and Yang

Olives nourish qi and blood. They relieve sore throat and dryness in the bronchi and lungs—keep an olive under your tongue when suffering from a sore throat. Olive counteracts alcoholism. An olive and ginger decoction will relieve dysentery and diarrhea.

Green: Protein, 1.5 g; Fat, 13.5 g; Fiber, 1.2 g; Carbohydrate, 4 g; Vitamin A, 300 IU; Vitamin B$_1$, traces; Vitamin B$_2$, traces; Niacin, traces; Vitamin C, traces; Calcium, 87 mg; Phosphorus, 17 mg; Iron, 1.6 mg

Black: Protein, 1.8 g; Fat, 21 g; Fiber, 1.5 g; Carbohydrate, 2.6 g; Vitamin A, 60 IU; Vitamin B$_1$, traces; Vitamin B$_2$, traces; Niacin, traces; Vitamin C, traces; Calcium, 87 mg; Phosphorus, 17 mg; Iron, 1.6 mg

Pepper (black and white)
Pungent (Metal), hot, Yang

Pepper has a strong warming effect on the stomach and intestines; it is therefore useful in clearing digestive and abdominal problems due to cold syndromes. Five or six corns of black pepper, ground and mixed with honey or brewed in a tea, are an aid to good digestion. Pepper should, however, be steered away from in summer or when suffering from hot- and dry-syndrome diseases.

White pepper is just black pepper without the skin. It has the same warming effects as black but is slightly more irritating to the taste buds. For medicinal purposes, white pepper is used more frequently than black.

Black: Protein, 4 g; Fat, 2 g; Fiber, –; Carbohydrate, 28 g; Vitamin A, 80 IU; Vitamin B$_1$, 0 mg; Vitamin B$_2$, 0.2 mg; Niacin, 0 mg; Vitamin C, –; Calcium, 180 mg; Phosphorus, 80 mg; Iron, 12.2 mg

White: Protein, 6 g; Fat, 2 g; Fiber, –; Carbohydrate, 34 g; Vitamin A, –; Vitamin B$_1$, 0 mg; Vitamin B$_2$, 0 mg; Niacin, 0 mg; Vitamin C, –; Calcium, 120 mg; Phosphorus, 80 mg; Iron, 6.8 mg

Pepper (red or cayenne)
Pungent (Metal), hot, Yang

Red pepper exerts a strong heating effect on the body, thus stimulating the heart, the spleen, the stomach, and all the digestive processes. It is believed in many countries, including China, that the consumption of cayenne pepper lowers cholesterol in the blood and therefore protects against heart disease. The consumption of red pepper is also said to soften the blood vessels, thereby alleviating arteriosclerosis and hypertension. Red pepper is useful as a disinfectant in hot climates, where bacteria thrive and can spoil fresh food in a matter of hours.

Protein, 4 g; Fat, 6 g; Fiber, –; Carbohydrate, 20 g; Vitamin A, 14,000 IU; Vitamin B$_1$, 0.2 mg; Vitamin B$_2$, 0.4 mg; Niacin, 4 mg; Vitamin C, 20 mg; Calcium, 60 mg; Phosphorus, 100 mg; Iron, 2.8 mg

Salt
Salty (Water), cold, Yin

Salt, like sugar, has received a lot of bad press in the West: salt leads to edema; it also hardens the arteries and increases blood pressure. Its consumption has been linked to heart disease and thrombosis. Salt, however, can also serve useful therapeutic purposes. Taken in small doses, it stimulates the kidneys and facilitates the functions of the abdominal organs. It softens hardened glands and muscles. It has a cooling effect on the blood, and serves to maintain cellular health.

In China, salt is commonly used as a remedy against abdominal pains. It can either be added to an equal quantity of rice wine and swallowed in one gulp, or it can be heated and pressed against the abdomen in a towel. Salt is also used as a cure for athlete's foot and, when drunk with water, as a remedy for constipation. Drinking large quantities of salt water is a quick way to induce vomiting in cases of food poisoning. Finally, salt is used in China as a mouthwash and oral cavity disinfectant. When no toothpaste is at hand, it is common to brush one's teeth with salt instead.

As is the case with sugar, refined salt (virtually pure sodium chloride) is less advisable than rock or sea salt. The latter contains useful "impurities" such as iodine that are beneficial to health. Refined salt contains no nutrients.

Seaweed
Salty (Water), cold, Yin

All varieties of seaweed are a good remedy for goiter because of their high iodine contents. Seaweed is also used in Chinese medicine for curing hypertension and as an expectorant for chronic bronchitis. Seaweed is rich in minerals that it absorbs from the sea bottom and is therefore a general tonic for all physical and mental functions. It is important to point out, however, that the seaweed must come from a nonpolluted seabed. Seaweed is an important part of people's diet in the coastal Zhejiang province of China. Being a highly industrialized area, many pollutants are discarded directly into the sea. It may not be a coincidence, therefore, that there is an extremely high correlation (82%) in Zhejiang province between rectal cancer and the consumption of sea vegetables.[13]

Fresh: Protein, 1.7 g; Fat, 0.6 g; Fiber, 0 g; Carbohydrate, 9.6 g; Vitamin A, 116 IU; Vitamin B_1, 0.05 mg; Vitamin B_2, 0.15 mg; Niacin, 0.5 mg; Vitamin C, 20 mg; Calcium, 168 mg; Phosphorus, 42 mg; Iron, 2.85 mg

Dried: Protein, 8.5 g; Fat, 3.0 g; Fiber, 0 g; Carbohydrate, 48 g; Vitamin A, 580 IU; Vitamin B_1, 0.25 mg; Vitamin B_2, 0.75 mg; Niacin, 2.5 mg; Vitamin C, 100 mg; Calcium, 840 mg; Phosphorus, 210 mg; Iron, 14.25 mg

Soy sauce
Sweet and salty (Earth and Water), thermally neutral, Yang

Soy sauce is used principally as a flavor enhancer. Because of its high sodium content, the excessive use of soy sauce can be deleterious to health. Sodium is known to harden the arteries and to increase blood pressure, however it is also added to food as an aid to digestion.

Soy sauce is commonly used as an application to alleviate the pain from bee or wasp stings; in the Chinese countryside it is sprinkled or lightly daubed on burns.

Protein, 2 g; Fat, 0 g; Fiber, 0 g; Carbohydrate, 4 g; Vitamin A, 15 IU; Vitamin B_1, 0.11 mg; Vitamin B_2, 0.05 mg; Niacin, 0.5 mg; Vitamin C, 3 mg; Calcium, 10 mg; Phosphorus, 45 mg; Iron, 0.38 mg

Vinegar
Sour and bitter (Wood and Fire),
warm, weak Yin

Chinese vinegar is usually made from rice, wheat, or sorghum. Vinegar stimulates the circulation of the blood, aids digestion, increases appetite, and detoxifies.

Studies conducted at the Research Institute of Epidemic Diseases at the Chinese Academy of Science in Beijing indicate that vinegar acts as a disinfectant. Using vinegar in this way, many people boil vinegar in the home during winter to guard against catching colds or the flu; many rural northern Chinese homes smell quite strongly of vinegar. This same method of boiling vinegar is used in higher dosage to arouse somebody who has fainted. Vinegar is frequently prescribed to treat hepatitis.

Vinegar has no nutritive value.

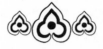

Chapter 5

CHINESE HOME REMEDIES FOR COMMON HEALTH CONDITIONS

Chinese medicine does not generally make clear distinctions between home remedies and official pharmacopoeia. Drugs and food merge in many preparations; however, drugs on their own can never take the place of food.

Most of the remedies in this chapter are food cures. They can be taken over long periods of time for daily nutrition as well as for curing ailments. Many can be taken regularly, even every day, for the rest of your life. If you tend to suffer from constipation, for example, there is no harm in eating two soft, very ripe bananas every morning and evening from now to eternity. However, although none of the remedies will produce ill side effects, a few are nonetheless best taken for short periods only. It would be rash, for example, to eat twenty egg yolks every day (a remedy for dysentery) or to consume bitter apricot kernels (a medium-grade drug in Chinese terms; see page 38) for more than two weeks at a time. Some remedies by nature are not to be taken for too long. This fact will be pointed out both in the written text and by means of the symbol 🖐.

At all times, simply use common sense and maintain a generally balanced diet for your body type and the time of year. Don't stick to a hot ginger cure for asthma, for example, if it's the middle of summer and you have a heat rash. The ginger will only make matters worse. Cure the acute problem first and return to your long-term therapy afterward.

When curing problems, one danger that you must always beware of is that of "treating the head when the head aches, treating the foot when the foot hurts," that is, treating the symptoms but not the disease. As you diagnose your condition, don't be superficial. Take a little time to wonder why you are suffering from something as seemingly innocuous as indigestion: was it the cold, too much to eat, or something specific in your food? What brought on your latest asthma attack? See a doctor first and listen to his or her diagnosis, then decide upon an appropriate Chinese food cure.

Occasionally you may come across recipes containing some particularly unpleasant ingredient—nothing toxic or dangerous, but not particularly palatable either. These recipes are described more for their authenticity than for practical purposes, although there is no harm in trying them if you wish to. As well, while traditional Chinese medicine tends toward ingestion of food or herbs as the primary remedy, sometimes massage, skin applications, or insertion of medicaments into orifices (such as garlic drops in the nostrils to cure a runny nose) are suggested. Where feasible, we have included these under the appropriate health problem.

Don't expect miracles. A natural cure always involves a slow process of fine adjustments. It takes time for the body to get out of balance, and time to get back in balance again. Patience is of the essence.

❖ ❖ ❖

Most of the remedies described in the following pages are straightforward and simple to prepare. No special expertise is necessary. Nevertheless, a few traditional aspects of preparation may be helpful to define.

COOKWARE

In China we traditionally steam rice and vegetables in earthenware, and stir-fry in an iron *guo* (in English, a "wok"). While these are still considered to be the best utensils, today enameled and stainless steel vessels are used as well. As far as we know there are no health hazards in using any of this cookware. Aluminum, however, may be less safe. Medical evidence links aluminum to Alzheimer's disease (senile dementia); heavy deposits of this metal are found on the brain synapses of Alzheimer's patients. It is not yet known whether aluminum causes Alzheimer's disease or whether the disease encourages the mineral to deposit. Until we know more conclusively, it may be preferable to stay away from aluminum foil and cooking utensils altogether, especially for preparations using acid foods, such as lemon, onion, tomato, or vinegar.[1] The acid tends to corrode, and thus carries more aluminum molecules into the body.

METHODS OF PREPARATION

Chopping

Chop your ingredients manually. Traditionalists claim that if you use a blender, the cutting speed and the heat generated will destroy many of the food's essential characteristics. The point is arguable, but there is, we believe, a psychological advantage to manually preparing your ingredients, as it involves time and attention and active care for the process of healing. If it is true that half our battles with illness are won or lost on psychosomatic grounds, spending time to wash, prepare, and concoct our medications by hand will put us in a more receptive frame of mind for taking them than if we simply swallow what an appliance machinates.

Grinding

Grind manually using a stone pestle. An alternative would be to grate the raw food, if appropriate.

Crushing

You can crush garlic, ginger, and onion by pressing down firmly on the food with the blade of a wide knife. Crushing makes the juice of the food more available.

Shredding

Shredding meat makes it more tender when cooked. To shred, first cut the meat into wide slices against the grain of the long muscle fibers. Then stack the slices and cut in the opposite direction. The pieces should end up being about 2 inches (5 centimeters) long and ¼ inch (6 millimeters) wide.

Squeezing Juice

While using a juicer is obviously the easiest way to obtain a food's liquid, it has the same drawbacks as using a blender for chopping. The traditional way to squeeze juice out of fruits, roots, and vegetables is to first either grate or chop the raw food into small pieces, then put it in a thin, clean cotton cloth. Squeeze by forming a bundle and tightening the cloth, twisting it in a viselike manner to extract the liquid.

Steaming

In China we have been steaming food for at least eight thousand years: the oldest cooking pots found in Neolithic villages in the Yellow River basin are terra-cotta steamers.[2] Steaming is one of the healthiest ways of cooking food. Frying alters a food's chemical composition, and boiling it causes many of the minerals and vitamins to be lost in the water. Steaming, on the other hand, best retains the food's color and nutritional value.

In order to steam you will need a large pot and a bamboo (or metal) steamer. Traditional Chinese steamers are round bamboo baskets that fit one on top of the other, thus enabling you to steam several dishes at the same time. If one or more of your ingredients are liquid, you will also need a ceramic bowl that fits into the steamer.

Place the food that you want to steam inside the steaming dish. Pour enough water into the bottom of the pot to produce steam for as long as your food cooks, then place the steamer containing your ingredients inside the pot. The steamer must fit comfortably, as there needs to be enough room for steam to circulate freely around the food; make sure, however, that the steamer is seated high enough that the boiling water will not come in contact with the food. Cover the pot with a tight-fitting lid.

In order to steam successfully, the water in the pot must actively boil. The steam from anything less than rapidly boiling water will not be sufficient to cook your food. You generally know the food is ready when you can smell it in the steam escaping from the lid.

Stir-frying

Although not generally a mode of preparation for food remedies, stir-frying is a common means of Chinese food preparation. Use a guo, referred to in English as a wok, or an ordinary frying pan. The guo or frying pan should be large enough to make stirring easy.

Use very little oil when stir-frying. In China we use peanut, corn, rape, or sunflower oil. Olive oil has recently become popular as well. Traditionally, sesame oil is considered high-quality oil, and black sesame oil is considered to be the best of all. Sesame oil is precious however, and these days is expensive. It was traditionally used only as a condiment in any but the imperial kitchens of old.

For vegetable dishes you may dispense with oil altogether. Use a nonstick guo, or use a little water instead of oil.

Cut your ingredients into pieces small enough to be cooked in 1 to 3 minutes. Use high heat and stir constantly.

Roasting

Roasting is a process of heating foods in a frying pan or wok without using either oil or water. Heat until the ingredient is dry and begins to brown on the outside. This procedure is frequently required for ingredients that need to be ground into a powder.

Decocting

To this day, medicinal decoctions are prepared exclusively in earthenware pots. These are specially designed crocks with a handle and spout. No household in China is complete without one.[3]

To prepare a decoction, wash and chop the ingredients. Add water and boil over a low to medium flame for 10 to 15 minutes. (Specific measurements and times will be given in the recipes.) Unless otherwise instructed, always cover the pan to keep the essential oils and other active ingredients from escaping into the air. Allow to cool, then drink the decoction warm or at room temperature. If you wish to, you may eat the boiled ingredients.

Storing

Unless specified in the recipes that follow, no preparation should be kept for more than a few days. Freshness assures that all the food's healing properties are intact. You may extend the life of your food remedy by putting it in the refrigerator (but not the freezer). Make sure, though, that you do not consume it refrigerator-cold; always allow it to reach room temperature before ingesting. Reheat gently if the remedy is to be taken hot.

SPECIAL INGREDIENTS

Vinegar

The traditional vinegar of Chinese medicine and cuisine is derived from rice. (Rice vinegar can be found these days in most health food stores.) Any vinegar made from fruits or cereals will do, however apple cider vinegar or red grape wine vinegar are among the best.

Wine

In China, *wine* usually refers to "rice spirit," or *sake* as it is generally known in America.[4] Sorghum or bamboo spirit is also used. What is important in Chinese recipes is not so much the flavor or origin of the wine but its light warming and rising effects. Many liquor stores stock sake and Chinese rice wine, though if you cannot find it, any wine or spirit will do.

Ginger

Ginger is one of the most important ingredients in Chinese healing cuisine. Although ginger has been exported to the West since the first century A.D., this pungent rhizome is native to southeast Asia and China, where it has been used as a flavoring, a spice, a food, a mouth cleanser, and a medicine since ancient times. The medicinal uses of ginger are many. Ginger stimulates the lungs, the stomach, and the spleen. Ginger has sweat-inducing (diaphoretic) qualities that render it a useful remedy for the common cold and influenza. It relieves nausea. A slice of ginger or some ginger juice will suppress motion sickness. Ginger combats indigestion and flatulence. It is also a strong anticoagulant; a few slices of this rhizome can guard against blood clots, and thus help prevent heart attack or thrombosis.

Ginger may be taken either fresh or dry.* Most of the recipes in this book that include ginger state that it should be fresh. Raw, fresh ginger exerts a milder effect than the dry rhizome; it is also easier to come by in supermarkets. Except when the remedy calls for squeezing the ginger for its juice, you may, if you wish, use dry ginger instead. Where fresh ginger only warms, dried ginger is stronger, more pungent, and has a heating and diaphoretic effect on the body. You may therefore want to take dry ginger for the extra punch, and in winter.

Rice

Rice grows all over China; each area has its own favorite variety. The most commonly used Chinese rices are similar to basmati or Thai jasmine rice. You can use either of those rices for all the recipes in this book. Both basmati and Thai jasmine rice can be found at natural foods stores.

Rice congee is simply overboiled white rice. To prepare a congee, put 1 cup of rice and 5 cups of water in a saucepan, over a medium-high flame. No salt, stock, or spice of any kind is added. When the water boils, turn the heat to medium; cover the pan and simmer for 20 minutes, stirring occasionally lest the rice stick to the bottom of the pan. The rice is boiled until it is soft and mushy. If necessary, add water every now and then so that you end up with a watery gruel.

Dried Flowers and Leaves

Several medicinal remedies in this chapter use dried chrysanthemum flowers, rose petals, and other plant parts. What you can't collect in the outdoors close to your home you can likely pick up at a Chinese grocer. Such plant preparations will sometimes be packaged as tea.

Bitter Apricot Kernel

As discussed on page 38, bitter apricot kernel is somewhat toxic and is thus considered a medium-grade drug in Chinese pharmacology. Bitter apricot kernel

---

* Dried ginger as referred to in these recipes is still in root form; it is not powdered. Dried ginger is used a lot in Chinese medicine. It is available at Chinese pharmacies.

is used to relieve cough, and as a treatment for asthma and acute or chronic bronchitis. It should not be eaten raw, or consumed for more than ten consecutive days. You can find bitter apricot kernel in Chinese pharmacies.

Bitter Melon

Bitter melon looks like a cucumber, but the color of the skin is much lighter. You can find bitter melon in Chinese groceries and in some supermarkets. Before cooking, split the melon lengthwise and discard the white part in the middle of the fruit.

Rock Sugar

Rock sugar, sometimes called rock candy, is sold in Chinese groceries. It is light brown in color and is less refined than the white rock sugar sold in candy stores.

❖ ❖ ❖

Having discussed the special ingredients and basic methods of preparation, we are now ready to look at many common ailments and health conditions that can be successfully treated with Chinese food and home remedies. We have listed these health conditions alphabetically. After a brief discussion of the problem from the point of view of both Chinese and Western medicine, we describe the remedies—the remedies are loosely grouped according to their main ingredients. The ingredient lists use standard measures, with approximate metric equivalents following in parentheses. We show the relative ease of preparation of the remedy, and the availability of the ingredients, by means of the following symbols.

Key to Symbols

👌👌👌	Easy recipe; can be prepared in a matter of minutes.
👌👌	Medium difficulty; takes a little time to prepare.
👌	A complex recipe that takes time and a little effort to prepare.
✍	All ingredients can be purchased with ease.
✍	Some of the ingredients may be difficult to find. You may have to go to a Chinese merchant in your area, or mail order the ingredients. An address list of select Chinese grocers willing to fill mail orders is given in appendix 2.
✋	Not recommended over long periods. Some ingredients are either bad for the health if taken for too long, or are slightly toxic (a second- or third-grade drug according to the Chinese classification of toxicity; see page 35).

ABDOMINAL PAINS

Abdominal pains are the physician's nightmare. They can have as many causes as there are diseases, ranging from cold to cancer. They may arise from the muscles of the abdomen, or from the diaphragm, the stomach, the spleen, the gallbladder, the large or small intestines, the appendix, the kidneys, the liver, or the nervous system. Consequently we cannot offer any remedies for abdominal pains without the risk of treating one problem for another, and thus bypassing the real cause altogether.

What we can do, and what the Chinese do before resorting to professional medical help, is to attribute the pains to the simplest possible causes and to take appropriate remedial action. If the pain persists, then you go to the doctor.

The simplest causes for abdominal pain are pathogenic cold (in Chinese terms), blocked digestion of food, and psychological distress.

Pathogenic cold can take hold of the body by two means: by simply catching cold, or by overeating raw or cold food ("cold" in both senses of the word: either direct from the refrigerator, or cold by nature). The symptoms of pathogenic cold are strong, cramplike pains; scanty and runny stools; cold feet and hands; and feeling repulsed by anything cold. A condition arising from pathogenic cold is relieved when the abdomen is covered and warmed.

Abdominal pains from blocked digestion are accompanied by heartburn, indigestion, and lack of appetite; you may also have diarrhea. Going to the toilet relieves the abdominal pain. Poor digestion may also be due to a weak stomach and/or spleen. If this is the case, it manifests as abdominal cramps that grow worse when you are overtired or hungry.

Psychological distresses—such as anger, worry, and frustration—block the free flow of zheng qi through the body. This is said to weaken the liver, spleen, and stomach, with consequent bloating and tummy pains.

Remedies for cold-syndrome abdominal pains require the ingestion of hot or warming foods. It also pays to cover the affected area with woolens.

Salty Wine

👍👍👍✋

3 tablespoons (45 mililiters) rice wine, or sake
5 teaspoons (25 grams) salt

In a small saucepan, heat the wine with the salt until the salt melts.
Drink hot—a single shot is generally sufficient.

Garlic and Ginger Broth

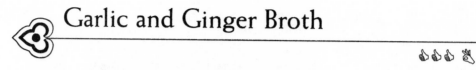

2 garlic cloves, peeled and crushed
2 teaspoons (10 grams) minced fresh or dry ginger
4 teaspoons (20 grams) brown sugar
2 cups (500 milliliters) water

Combine all ingredients in a small saucepan. Boil for 15 minutes over a low flame.

Drink the broth hot to warm, as often as you'd like. Eat the garlic and ginger pieces.

Garlic Tea

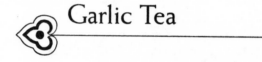

5 whole garlic cloves, peeled
2 cups (500 milliliters) water
1 tablespoon (15 grams) brown sugar or
    molasses (15 mililiters)

Combine the ingredients in a small saucepan. Boil for 15 minutes over a low flame. Remove from heat.

Drink 1 cup three times a day, following a meal. Prepare fresh on each occasion.

Ginger Vinegar

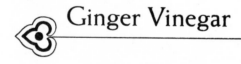

In many Chinese homes, a bottle of ginger vinegar is always at hand for emergency treatment of abdominal pains.

$\frac{1}{2}$ cup (100 grams) fresh ginger, thinly sliced
1 cup (250 milliliters) rice wine vinegar

Place the ginger and vinegar together in a bottle. Cap the bottle and store. (The longer the vinegar is stored the better. Ideally you should leave it for a month, but a few hours will do in an emergency.)

Take 2 teaspoons every morning on an empty stomach.

Sometimes garlic is added for a richer brew: the proportions are ½ cup (100 grams) of ginger, ½ cup (100 grams) of garlic, and 2 cups (500 milliliters) of vinegar. The garlic cloves should be whole when added to the vinegar. Besides curing abdominal ailments caused by cold, ginger and garlic vinegar counteracts abdominal pains resulting from eating too much fruit.

Garlic Vinegar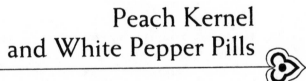

👍👍✌️

12 whole garlic cloves, peeled
1 cup (250 milliliters) rice vinegar

Place the garlic cloves and vinegar together in a bottle. Cap tightly and store. Take 2 teaspoons every morning on an empty stomach, or as needed.

In the Chinese countryside some people store vinegar for two or three years before consuming. For a "fast food" version, however, one month is adequate. Garlic vinegar remedies cold pains as well as those due to psychological distress and an irregular lifestyle. (One wonders whether it is the garlic vinegar that cures the pains or just waiting for it that cures the lifestyle.)

Peach Kernel and White Pepper Pills

👍👍🖌️

5 peach seeds
5 jujube (Chinese date)
8 white peppercorns

Break open the peach seeds and remove the kernels. Using a stone grinder or a pestle, manually crush the kernels together with jujube and peppercorns. Compress into swallowable pills.

Ingest with warm rice wine or warm red wine.

Cinnamon Water

1 teaspoon (5 grams) ground cinnamon
1 glass warm water

Dissolve the cinnamon in the water. Drink slowly.

To be effective, this remedy should be taken three times a day.

Cinnamon exerts a warming effect that is also useful in alleviating abdominal pains after childbirth. Again, drink 1 teaspoon of ground cinnamon dissolved in warm water three times a day.

For cramps and muscular pains in the abdominal region, whatever the cause, the following remedies are recommended.

Sesame, Walnut, and Ginger Paste

³/₄ cup (150 grams) sesame seeds
³/₄ cup (150 grams) walnut meats
³/₄ cup (150 grams) dried ginger, chopped
³/₄ cup (185 milliliters) honey

Grind the sesame seeds, walnuts, and ginger into a medium-grained powder. It is preferable to use either a stone grinder or a pestle. Roast the powder in a dry frying pan or wok for 2 minutes, or until it begins to brown. Transfer the powder to a small bowl. Mix with the honey while still hot.

Take ¹/₂ cup (100 grams) of paste on an empty stomach whenever you suffer from abdominal cramps and pains.

Hot Salt Compress

👍👍👍 ✌️

When suffering from abdominal pains due to cold syndrome it is best to warm the affected area—the Chinese recommend wearing woolen clothes or wraps. You can also press a hot towel or muslin bag containing heated salt over your abdomen. You might want to try this when it is very cold, or if your pains are particularly bad.

1 cup (250 grams) rock salt
Dry cloth towel or muslin bag

Heat the salt in a dry frying pan or wok. When the salt starts to crack, transfer it to a dry towel or cloth bag. (If you are using a towel, fold it to create a pouch for containing the salt.)

Apply to your abdomen for five to ten minutes while lying down. Repeat three times a day. (You can use the same salt.) See also the salt and onion application recommended for diarrhea, page 132.

ACNE

Acne, an inflammation of the skin, affects 80 percent of people during adolescence and early adulthood. Acne occurs when oil from the sebaceous glands gets trapped under the skin, causing bacteria to multiply. The result is inflammation and pustules. Contributory factors to acne are oily skin (which may be hereditary), excessive male hormones, allergies, oral contraceptives, stress, alcohol, sugar, and junk food.

According to Chinese traditional medicine, acne is usually due to one of two possible causes: excessive heat in the lungs and stomach, or external cold interacting with too many alcoholic beverages. (Many Chinese are sturdy drinkers.) In the latter case the blood is said to "silt up"; the nose and the cheeks redden. Finally, the face erupts with acne. The complaint is worsened by psychological tension.

To treat acne, Western and Chinese doctors alike recommend that you avoid fat foods, sweets, and alcohol, and that you wash your face morning and evening with a mild, alkaline-free soap. Do not overwash—this will stimulate an overproduction of sebum as the body tries to replenish its lost oils. Lemon or lime juice can also be used for cleansing. In China, where lemons are not common, other ingredients are used for washing. These include:

◆ Mix celery and apple juice together in equal quantities. Apply to the face morning and evening.
◆ Cut a water chestnut in half. Rub the inside cross-section over your face two or three times a day.
◆ As soon as you wake up, apply your own saliva to the area affected by acne. When the saliva dries, apply again. Repeat throughout the morning.

Two simple food remedies for acne include eating plenty of raw cucumber, which exerts a cooling effect on the stomach and lungs, and drinking large quantities of hot green tea.

To finish, a simple recipe follows.

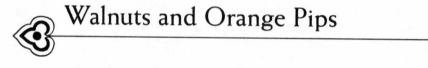

Walnuts and Orange Pips

2 walnuts, shelled
1 tablespoon (15 grams) dried orange seeds (you might wish to roast the orange seeds slightly in order to hasten the drying process)

Using a stone grinder or pestle, grind the walnuts and orange seeds into a fine powder. Roast in a dry wok for 2 or 3 minutes over low flame, or until the powder begins to brown. Remove the wok from the heat and allow the powder to cool.

Take all the powder with a small amount of rice wine twice a day.

ALCOHOLISM

Although it has been demonstrated that small doses of alcohol have dilative and cholesterol-cleansing effects on the arteries and veins, large quantities of alcohol are poisonous.

Short-term alcohol poisoning—otherwise known as inebriation—may cloud the intellect with temporary euphoria. Other effects such as slower reaction times, speaking incoherently, unsteadiness, and the morning-after hangover may be less welcome.

Long-term alcohol poisoning causes metabolic damage to every cell in the body. It brings about rapid aging, increases susceptibility to disease, and generally shortens one's life span by several years. Alcohol is broken down in the liver, where it is converted into fat; ironically, at the same time as it is being broken down by the liver it is destroying the cells of the liver. A damaged liver impairs metabolism and the processes of digestion and absorption of proteins and vitamins. In short, dependency on alcohol, be it physical or psychological, kills.

Although short-term alcohol abuse in China is fairly common, chronic alcoholism is not. People drink in short, hard bursts rather than out of habit. Liquor—usually rice wine—is quaffed at banquets and during celebrations. People drink when reciting poetry, or as a competitive game to see who gets drunk first. As a consequence, Chinese culture has many popular remedies for drunkenness, but none, besides sheer willpower, for chronic alcoholism.

There are several food cures in China for recovering a modicum of lucidity when drunk.

- ❖ The most common remedy for inebriation is to drink a cup of strong black tea; strong jasmine tea also works. Brew the tea as usual; just put more leaves in the pot. Strong tea tastes quite bitter. The sobering effect is enhanced if you do not add sugar.
- ❖ Radish juice and vinegar is another common remedy for inebriation. Squeeze ¹/₂ cup (125 milliliters) of fresh radish juice, then add 1 teaspoon (5 milliliters) of vinegar. Swallow the mixture in one gulp.
- ❖ An easy remedy is to crush 1 raw sweet potato and add sugar. Mix with hot water and drink.
- ❖ A quick remedy, if you happen to live in the tropics, is to drink a glass of green sugarcane juice.
- ❖ As a preventive measure, it is alleged that eating a persimmon before going on a drinking binge will prevent the ill effects of alcohol.

Some recipes requiring a little more preparation follow.

Mung Bean Soup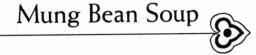

👍👍 ✋

¹/₄ cup (50 grams) green mung beans
1 cup (250 milliliters) cold water

Grind the mung beans into a fine powder using a stone grinder or a pestle. Transfer the powder to a glass.

Add water and mix. Drink immediately.

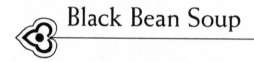

Tea and Mung Beans

👍👍👌

> 1/4 cup (50 grams) mung beans
> 1 teaspoon (5 grams) green tea leaves
> 2 cups (500 milliliters) water

Roast the mung beans in a dry frying pan or wok until they begin to brown. Allow the beans to cool, then grind them into a powder using a stone grinder or a pestle.

Bring the water to a boil. Put the mung bean powder into a teapot or large cup. Add tea leaves and hot water. Cover the teapot or cup, and steep for 10 minutes.

Drink hot, without sugar.

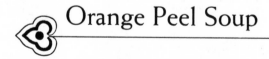

Black Bean Soup

👍👍👍👌

> 4 cups (800 grams) black beans
> 8 cups (2 liters) water

In a soup kettle or large saucepan, boil black beans and water for 45 minutes. Keep the pan uncovered. The mixture will become quite thick as it boils. Check occasionally to make sure that it is not so thick that it begins to dry and burn; add a little water if necessary.

When the beans are done, take the pot off the stove and allow the mixture to cool. Drain, reserving the beans for another use.

Drink the soup, continuing until you throw up.

Orange Peel Soup

👍👍👌

> The peel of 1 organic orange
> 2 cups (500 milliliters) water
> 1/3 teaspoon (1.5 grams) salt

In a dry frying pan, roast the orange peel over medium heat until it turns light brown. Cool and grind to a powder.

In a small saucepan, combine orange peel powder, water, and salt. Boil for thirty minutes, covered.

Drink hot to warm.

Ginger Soymilk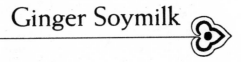

👍👍✍

2 teaspoons (10 grams) fresh or dry ginger, minced
1 cup (250 milliliters) soymilk
2 tablespoons (30 grams) rock sugar

Put all the ingredients into a small saucepan. Bring to a boil; continue to boil for 10 minutes.

Remove from heat and allow to cool slightly. Drink warm.

ANEMIA

Anemia results from a reduction of red blood corpuscles and, as a consequence, of the amount of oxygen that the blood is able to carry. Its early symptoms are poor appetite, dizziness, constipation, irritability, ringing in the ears, and headaches. Anemia is characterized by general fatigue and debility, and by pallid nails and inner eyelids.

Anemia is not a common ailment in China. Indeed, one quite surprising fact to emerge from a 1991 survey of Chinese diet, lifestyle, and mortality was that iron intake is much higher in China than in the United States.[5] The reason for the difference puzzled the researchers, as the intake of iron-rich foods seems no higher in China than in America. Leaching of iron from food containers was not considered likely because such containers are not generally used in food storage. A tentative suggestion put forward by the researchers was that iron may simply be absorbed through dust; another possibility is the use of the traditional iron guo (wok) in food preparation. Nothing has been steadfastly agreed upon.

Despite its rarity, anemia is divided by traditional Chinese medicine into three categories:

1. Anemia resulting from a lack of iron in the diet.
2. Anemia brought on by loss of blood from wounds, heavy menstruation, an ulcer, or hemorrhoids.
3. Anemia caused by bone marrow disease, a damaged liver, a thyroid disorder, or rheumatoid arthritis.

Given these variations, whenever anemia is suspected a professional consultation to discover the underlying cause is mandatory.

Temporary, nonpathological anemia can be easily cured by increasing the intake of iron. Iron makes hemoglobin, which carries oxygen in the blood.

Good natural sources of iron are apricots, jujube (Chinese dates), beets, grapes, lettuce, cashews, honey, blackstrap molasses, soybeans, and spinach. Liver and raw liver extract contain the elements essential for reconstituting the red blood cells. Iron tablets, an effective cure for temporary anemia, tend to cause constipation. Tannic acid, present in tea and coffee, and dairy products inhibit the absorption of iron. Vitamin C assists its absorption.

Some food remedies for anemia are quite simple.

- ❖ You can take 2 or 3 tablespoons (30 to 45 milliliters) of honey a day in any form: in warm water, with your breakfast cereal, on toast, or on its own.
- ❖ Another remedy is to tear 1 small fig leaf into strips, then decoct in 1 cup (250 milliliters) of boiling water. Drink the tea.
- ❖ You can also grind peanut husks into a powder; take 1 heaping teaspoon twice a day with warm water.
- ❖ Mix 2 or 3 tablespoons (30 or 45 milliliters) of raw carrot juice with the same amount of molasses. Take twice a day.
- ❖ It is also widely believed that boiled eggs with tomatoes taken as a salad two or three times a day, and 1 apple, 1 tomato, and 3 teaspoons of sesame seeds taken as a salad once or twice a day, will both cure anemia.

Recipes involving a bit more preparation include the following.

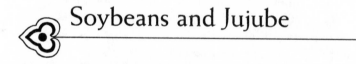

Soybeans and Jujube

1 tablespoon (15 grams) soybeans
Water for soaking
3 cups (750 milliliters) water
1 tablespoon (15 grams) jujube (Chinese dates)
1 tablespoon (15 grams) brown sugar

Soak the soybeans overnight in 1 cup (250 milliliters) of water. Drain.

In a medium saucepan, bring 1½ cups (325 milliliters) of water to boil. Add the drained beans and boil them for approximately 20 minutes. In a separate saucepan, bring the remaining 1½ cups (325 milliliters) of water to boil. Add the jujube and brown sugar. Boil for 10 minutes.

Add the jujube and their water to the black beans. Stir to mix.

Consume the entire soup warm, in one sitting. Take once a day; a full course of treatment lasts two weeks.

Tofu and Egg White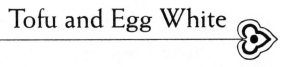

👍👍✌️

1 pound (500 grams) tofu, frozen
5 cups (1.25 liters) warm water
2 egg whites
Water for steaming

Place the frozen tofu in warm water. (Freezing tofu changes its texture, rendering it spongelike and thus capable of absorbing the egg white.) When the tofu has become soft, remove it from the water and transfer to a bowl holding the egg whites.

Soak the tofu in the egg whites for 5 minutes, then transfer to a large ceramic bowl. Put the bowl in a steaming dish (see page 66). Using a pot deep enough to fit your steamer, bring water to a boil. Put the steamer in the pot and cover. Steam the tofu for 15 minutes.

Remove from the steamer. Eat warm.

Liver and Spinach Stew

👍👍✌️

2 cups (500 milliliters) water
4 ounces (125 grams) calf's liver, cubed
½ pound (250 grams) fresh packed spinach

In a medium saucepan, bring the water to a boil. When the water boils, add the liver and spinach. Reduce heat to low and cover the pan.

Stew the mixture for 45 minutes. Check occasionally to ensure that the stew is not too dry; if necessary, add a little water.

Consume hot; eat the stew all at once. Take this remedy as often as you want.

Wood-ear Mushrooms and Jujube Dessert

¹/₄ cup (50 grams) wood-ear mushrooms (also known as
  tree ears)
Water for soaking
3 cups (750 milliliters) water
30 jujube (Chinese dates)
Brown sugar to taste

Soak the mushrooms in 1 cup (250 milliliters) of hot water for 1 hour, or until soft. Drain.

In a small saucepan, bring the water to a boil. Boil the mushrooms and jujube until the jujube are soft, approximately 20 minutes. Stir in the brown sugar.

Consume in a single sitting, either warm or at room temperature.

ARTHRITIS

Arthritis, one of the most common diseases in China, is characterized by an inflammation of the joints. Rheumatoid arthritis attacks the synovial membranes of the joints, while osteoarthritis affects the bones. Both diseases are degenerative and deforming, and eventually affect the mobility of the limbs and joints. Their causes are hereditary, although cold, humidity, a faulty diet, stress, and emotional repression contribute to worsening the effects of these problems.

According to traditional Chinese medicine, arthritis is caused by the exogenous pathogens, specifically those of feng (wind), han (cold), and shi (dampness). These enter the main and collateral channels of qi circulation, thereby disturbing normal functions. The results are pain or numbness, and swelling in the joints and limbs.

Chinese remedial therapies for arthritis are based on correcting the effects of cold and dampness in one's food intake and in the environment. A person with arthritis should thus stay away from cold and damp foods and environments, and refrain from consuming too much red meat, sugar and sugar products, milk, fats, acid fruits (oranges and lemons), salt, and tobacco. Direct therapies on the affected areas of the body consist of heat and drug application. Movement exercises focused on the affected area are also beneficial. In fact, the most common treatment in China for arthritic disease is qi gong combined with massage and, if possible, acupuncture. See chapter 7 for detailed instruction in qi gong. You should prepare for your exercises by breathing deeply in the qi gong standing position, arms outstretched, for ten to fifteen minutes. Qi gong exercises that specifically loosen the joints are the Eight Brocade *ba duan jin* series and *tai ji quan*. Hot baths and massage are also useful.

Theory alleges that you can cure a disease in your own body by eating the same body parts from a healthy animal. The classic Chinese remedies for arthritis consist of animals and animal parts, the consumption of which is not only abhorrent to most people in the Western world but is also cruel to the animals concerned. Some of the animals whose bones are so prized by many of China's arthritis patients are endangered; first and foremost of these endangered animals is the tiger.

Tiger and leopard bone and sinew have always been considered the prime remedy for arthritic diseases. Lip service is paid to protecting the animals, yet many Chinese texts still extol the virtues of tiger bone as a cure for arthritis. Tigers continue to be poached, their body parts openly sold in crowded markets.[6]

Because of the difficulty and expense involved in obtaining the prized tiger, it has now become common to use dog bones as an arthritis remedy instead. Sometimes the dog bones are sold fraudulently as tiger; however, most often there is no deception involved. People eat dog meat and consume dog-bone preparations in the belief that these products warm the body and rid it of the external pathogens responsible for arthritis.[7] (Lest some of our readers start getting ideas about their neighbor's bothersome dog, we shall not go into details of how these particular remedies are prepared.)

Deer antlers and tendons are other prized alternatives to tiger parts, as are pig, sheep, and monkey bones.

One recipe that, although unusual, we have few qualms about describing is snake soup. Although frequently seen in small countryside restaurants, particularly in the south of China, snake is not a common dish. It is considered something of an expensive delicacy, to be resorted to only for purposes of restoring good health. Snake meat has a delicate flavor, somewhere between that of chicken and fish. It is highly prized in China. Fresh snake blood and snake bile are drunk with rice spirit; they are said to augment qi and to reinforce the internal organs of digestion. Snake meat is normally eaten in a soup, with the bones included as part of the broth.

Dragon and Phoenix Soup

5 ounces (150 grams) snake meat, cut into 2-inch-long pieces
3½ ounces (100 grams) chicken breast, cut into narrow,
    2-inch-long pieces
¾ ounce (20 grams) ham, cut into narrow, 2-inch-long pieces
3½ ounces (100 grams) bamboo shoots, optional
4 cups (1 liter) water
5 slices fresh ginger
2 teaspoons (10 milliliters) cooking wine, optional
2 teaspoons (10 milliliters) sesame oil
Pepper and salt to taste

Place the meat and bamboo shoots in soup pot. Add water, ginger, and cooking wine (if desired). Cook over a low flame, covered, for 1 hour, or until the snake meat turns white. Add sesame oil, pepper, and salt.
    Serve warm.

Snake and Black Bean Soup

1 adult snake, the more venomous the better
⅓ cup (65 grams) black beans
5 slices fresh ginger
10 jujube (Chinese dates)
Water to cover
Salt to taste

In order not to risk snakebite, it is probably preferable to have a professional catch, kill, and skin the snake for you. If you must do it on your own, hold the snake firmly behind the head and away from your body. Cut its head off, being careful not to touch the severed head—the venom is still present and the snake can still bite through muscular contraction. Most people in China collect the snake's blood in a glass, add rice spirit, and drink it in a single gulp.
    Skin the snake and clean out the innards. Chop the snake meat into 2-inch-long segments.
    Place all the ingredients into a soup pot. Add enough water to cover. Put the lid on the pot. Cook on a medium flame for 1 hour, or until the beans are soft, stirring occasionally. Add salt according to taste.
    Serve as part of a several course meal.

Silkworm Excrement Wine

Perhaps the main problem with this recipe is obtaining silkworm excrement. If you do not live close to a silk-producing area, it is unlikely that you will come by any very easily. However the recipe is interesting, and if you ever happen to go to China, or to where silkworms are abundant, you might wish to try it. Silkworm excrement is said to rid the body of evil wind and dampness.

    3 to 4 tablespoons (45–60 grams) silkworm excrement
    2 cups (500 milliliters) water
    1 shot rice wine, or sake

Place the silkworm excrement in a cloth bag.

In a small saucepan, bring the water to a boil. Add the cloth bag. Cover the pan and continue to boil for 10 minutes.

Add the rice wine, cover the pan, and allow to boil for another minute. Remove from heat.

Divide the wine into three cups. Drink one cup in the morning, one in the afternoon, and one in the evening for as long as the pain persists.

A few more practical recipes for our less adventurous readers follow.

White Bean and Jujube Congee

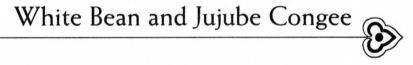

    4 tablespoons (60 grams) white black-eyed peas
    10–15 jujube (Chinese dates)
    2 tablespoons (30 grams) minced fresh ginger
    Scant $^1/_2$ cup (100 grams) rice
    4 cups (1 liter) water
    Salt or honey to taste

Put all the ingredients in a medium saucepan and bring to boil over a high flame. Turn the heat to low, cover the pot, and simmer for 30 minutes, or until the rice is soft and mushy. Stir occasionally.

Remove from heat. You may, if you wish to, add either salt or honey for flavor.

Eat whenever your joints are swollen or numb, either for breakfast or before bed.

Fresh Cherry Wine

2 cups (400 grams) fresh cherries
4 cups (1 liter) rice wine, or sake

Wash the cherries. When they are dry, place cherries in a bottle with rice wine. Seal the bottle.

Let stand to macerate for at least 15 days. When aged, take 2 teaspoons twice a day.

Tofu and Scallion

3¹⁄₂ ounces (100 grams) tofu
3 cups (750 milliliters) water
1 tablespoon (20 grams) minced scallions
1 teaspoon (5 milliliters) sesame oil
Soy sauce to taste

In a medium saucepan, bring the water to a boil. Drop the block of tofu into the water and cover the pan. Boil for 10 minutes, then drain.

Cut the boiled tofu into cubes. Season with scallions, sesame oil, and soy sauce. Consume warm.

This remedy should be eaten as part of a meal. Take as often as you want.

Stir-fried Bean Sprouts

1 tablespoon (15 milliliters) peanut oil
1 cup (200 grams) bean sprouts
1 tablespoon (15 milliliters) cooking wine
Salt to taste

Heat the oil in a wok or frying pan. When the oil is hot, add the bean sprouts. Stir-fry for 20 seconds, then add the wine and a little salt according to taste. Continue to stir-fry for 30 seconds. Remove from heat and serve.

This dish is generally served as part of a several course meal, and is eaten with rice.

Bean-thread Noodles and Cucumber

👍👍✌

1 cup (200 grams) bean-thread noodles
Water for soaking
2 cups (400 grams) cucumber, sliced
1 teaspoon (5 grams) salt
3 cups (750 milliliters) water
1 tablespoon (15 grams) minced scallions
3 tablespoons (45 milliliters) soy sauce
1 tablespoon (15 milliliters) vinegar
1–2 pinches white pepper
Salt to taste

Soak the bean-thread noodles in 2 cups (500 milliliters) of hot water for 10 minutes, or until soft. Drain.

In a small bowl, toss the cucumber slices with 1 teaspoon (5 grams) of salt. Let stand for 10 minutes to extract the cucumber juice. Drain.

In a medium saucepan, bring the water to a boil. Drop the bean thread in the boiling water. Boil for 5 minutes. Drain.

Mix the bean thread and cucumber with the scallions, soy sauce, vinegar, white pepper, and salt.

This dish may be eaten whenever your joints are swollen or feel hot.

The following are recipes for compresses to be used on inflamed joints.

Ginger and Vinegar Compress

👍👍👍✌

4 tablespoons (60 grams) sliced fresh ginger
1 cup (250 milliliters) rice vinegar
2 cups (500 milliliters) water

In a medium saucepan, bring all ingredients to boil over a high flame. Turn the flame to low. Simmer for 5 minutes.

Soak flannel cloths in the hot liquid. Remove the cloths; keeping the liquid simmering in the pot, let the cloths cool to the point that they can be handled. Apply the cloths to the affected body areas.

After the flannel cools, soak and apply again. After 5 or 10 minutes of compress application, massage those same areas of the body to which the cloths have been applied.

Apply twice daily—once in the morning and once in the evening.

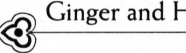 Scallion and Vinegar Compress

♨♨♨ ✌

4 tablespoons (60 grams) chopped scallions, white heads only
4 cups (1 liter) rice vinegar

In a medium saucepan boil the vinegar over a medium flame, uncovered, until half of it has evaporated. Add the chopped scallions to the vinegar and boil for another five minutes.

Turn the flame to low. Soak flannel cloths in the hot liquid. Let the cloths cool to the point that they are possible to touch, all the while keeping the liquid simmering in the pot. Apply the cloths to the affected body areas.

After the flannel cools, soak and apply again. After 5 or 10 minutes of applications, massage those same areas of the body.

Apply twice daily—once in the morning and once in the evening.

Ginger and Honey Compress

♨♨ ✌

2 tablespoons (30 grams) minced fresh ginger
¹/₃ cup (65 grams) taro root, peeled and sliced
¹/₃ cup (65 grams) white flour
2–3 tablespoons (30–45 milliliters) honey

Using a pestle, mash the ginger and the taro root into a fairly smooth paste. Transfer to a small bowl. Add the flour and 1 tablespoon (15 milliliters) of honey, mixing the ingredients by hand. Continue adding honey until you have a smooth paste.

Use a clean, dry cloth to collect the paste. Press to the painful joint or limb, and wrap.

Keep the wrap in place all day and night. Use for ten days to one month, changing the compress every 24 hours.

Chili Pepper and Ginger Compress

👍👍✌️

2 tablespoons (30 grams) chopped dried chili peppers
2 tablespoons (30 grams) chopped fresh or dried ginger
2 tablespoons (30 grams) white flour
2–3 tablespoons (30–45 milliliters) rice wine, or sake

In a small bowl, mix the chili peppers, ginger, and flour. Slowly pour the rice wine, or sake, over the dry ingredients, mixing to form a paste.

Apply the paste to the distressed joint or limb by means of a clean cotton cloth. Wrap or hold in place for half an hour, then wash with warm water and dry.

This compress may be applied twice a day, morning and evening, for as long as the discomfort persists.

ASTHMA

Asthma is generally hereditary in nature. It is characterized by attacks of coughing, wheezing, and gasping for breath. It is usually brought on by an allergic reaction to pollen, animal dander, mold spores, or foodstuffs. The only immediate remedy at the moment of an asthma attack is the administration of antihistamines such as epinephrine, and, in the most acute cases, of oxygen.

Chinese medicine tends to regard asthma as a weakness of the lungs brought about by climatic factors and worsened by poor eating habits and a stressful lifestyle. The first remedy, therefore, is to correct your errors.

The next obvious thing to do is stay away from the source of your allergy. If you are allergic to pollen or house dust, however, there is not a great deal you can do about it. In this case you should simply adopt the Chinese line of defense: get plenty of exercise; practice qi gong; stop smoking; do not fatigue yourself, either at work or in bed; and eat properly.

The latter advice includes eliminating unnecessary toxins from your diet by cutting down on (or dispensing altogether with) coffee, alcohol, strong tea, and fried and greasy food. Eat plenty of greens, fruits, beans, and cereals; eat less meat and few fats. Avoid hot, spicy, sour, salty, and very sweet foods. You should eat regular meals, never overindulging—get up from the dinner table knowing that you could eat a little more without stuffing yourself. Have dinner at least three hours before bedtime; eat slowly and chew properly. Drink plenty of water and fruit juices.

There are eight traditional Chinese remedies for asthma. Five are straightforward food remedies. One contains bitter apricot kernels (see page 69), which are slightly toxic; it must therefore be classified as a medicine rather than a food, and be taken for not more than ten days at a stretch. Another of the remedies for asthma involves the application of garlic to the sole of the foot. The last, involving fourteen eggs, has been practiced in China for centuries. We do not expect many people to try it, but have included it here because of its authenticity.

Many of the remedies for asthma use ginger as a main ingredient. Ginger is a warm and pungent tuber of the Jin (Metal) element. It is an outward- and upward-moving Yang ingredient that directly affects the lungs.

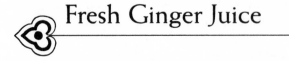

Fresh Ginger Juice

This remedy is particularly effective for older people with asthma.

16–20 ounces (500+ grams) fresh ginger, peeled and grated
8 tablespoons brown sugar

Place the grated ginger in a thin cotton towel. Squeeze to extract ½ cup of juice.

In a small saucepan, heat the ginger juice. Add the sugar, stirring until it dissolves. Bring the mixture just to the boiling point, then remove from heat and transfer to a cup.

Take this preparation while it is still hot, sipping slowly. Take it as long as the asthma persists.

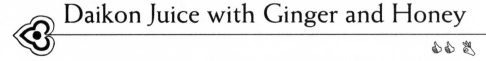

Daikon Juice with Ginger and Honey

1 4-ounce piece (125 grams) fresh ginger, peeled and grated
1 large fresh daikon, grated
2 tablespoons (30 milliliters) honey

Place the ginger and the daikon in separate thin cotton towels. Squeeze to extract 2 tablespoons of ginger juice and 1 cup of daikon juice.

Mix all ingredients in a small saucepan. Heat but do not boil.

Drink hot once a day.

Ginger and Rice Wine

Rice wine enhances the warming properties of ginger by making them rise toward the Yang (higher) regions of the body.

> **2 cups (400 grams) fresh ginger, sliced thin**
> **2 cups (500 milliliters) rice wine, or sake**
> **3 cups (600 grams) rock sugar**

Place the ginger in a medium saucepan with the rice wine. Bring to boil over a low flame. Add the sugar. Stir continuously as you simmer for another 20 to 30 minutes, until the mixture is a creamy paste.

Remove from heat and allow to cool.

Younger people can take 1 tablespoon with warm water every morning before breakfast during asthma season. Older adults and chronic asthma sufferers should increase the dosage to 1 tablespoon twice a day, before meals.

Ginger, Walnut, and Bitter Apricot Kernel Pills

This recipe uses bitter apricot kernels (see page 69), which are toxic when raw. It is therefore defined as a medium-grade drug in the Chinese classification of toxicity (see page 35). We have included it because of its efficacy in treating asthma. Be sure not to take it for more than ten days, and to wait at least three weeks before resuming the cure. The prescription should be taken during periods in which you normally suffer from asthma.

> **¹/₄ cup (50 grams) walnut meats**
> **¹/₄ cup (50 grams) bitter apricot kernels**
> **Water for soaking**
> **¹/₄ cup (50 grams) fresh ginger**
> **¹/₄ cup (60 milliliters) honey**

Soak the walnuts and bitter apricot kernels in water overnight, so as to be able to peel them with ease. Drain.

Peel the skin from the walnuts and the apricot kernels. Chop into fine pieces, together with the ginger. Transfer to a dry bowl. Mix with the honey to make a thick paste.

Roll the paste into 100 round pills. Take 10 pills a day for ten days, before going to bed.

Mud Orange

1 pound (500 grams) powdered clay (use soil if clay is not available)
1 cup (250 milliliters) water
1 orange

In a bowl, mix the clay or soil with water to form a thick paste. Pack the orange in the paste. Bake at 350°F for 10 minutes. Remove from the oven and allow to cool.

Wash the paste off the orange by holding it under running water. Split the orange open and eat the fruit while it is still warm.

To be taken once a day for seven days.

Garlic and Sugar

1 garlic clove, finely minced
2 tablespoons (30 grams) white sugar
1 small glass warm water

Mix the garlic with the sugar in the glass of warm water. Leave to brew for five minutes.

While the asthma is activated, take every evening before bed.

Garlic Foot Application

In this remedy, a clove of partially squeezed garlic is placed in the center of the sole of the foot, where the toe bones begin. This is an important point associated with the kidney channel. The lungs correspond to the Metal element, which generates Water (kidney) and subjugates Wood (liver). When the lungs are out of balance, as with asthma, the kidneys are directly affected.

2 garlic cloves
2 Band-Aids

Peel the garlic. Crush each clove slightly in order to crack it. Bind a clove to the middle of each sole, in the soft spot where the toe bones begin. Use a fresh clove of garlic every twenty-four hours.

Cured Eggs

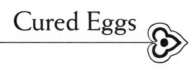

14 raw eggs, whole
Your own urine

Soak the raw eggs in the urine for seven days, changing the urine every twenty-four hours. Eat 2 eggs every morning, either raw or soft-boiled for 3 minutes. Continue the treatment for three months.

ATHLETE'S FOOT (TINEA PEDIS)

Athlete's foot is a fungus that thrives in warm, damp folds of skin between the toes. People who wear open sandals or no footwear at all rarely suffer from athlete's foot. However, if one lives in a warm, damp area and wears shoes, the perfect environment is created for this bothersome fungus to develop.

The most obvious preventive measures are to keep the feet aired and dry, and to change your socks and shoes every day. You can wear your shoes again five days later—the passage of time allows the shoes to air out. Get into the habit of rapidly passing the toes of your socks through the area when you put your socks on and when you remove them. Make sure that you dry the area with a towel after bathing or showering.

If, in spite of the preventive methods, you do catch the fungus, you can dab or spray perfume between the toes. Over-the-counter medications consist of zinc salt and undecylenic acid; compounds of this acid are present in perfumes.

Alcohol-based perfumes are not, however, common in China. Other methods have therefore been developed for dealing with athlete's foot.

- Salt renders an environment inhospitable to fungi. Take 6 pounds (2.7 kilos) of common salt. Place the salt in a dry saucepan and roast it for 10 minutes or until hot. Remove from the saucepan and place on a clean, dry towel. Fold the towel over the salt and place on the ground. Stand on the towel until the salt becomes cold. This should be done every day before bed, until you are rid of the problem.
- Apply a small amount of toothpaste between the toes three times a day.
- Take 4 cups (1 liter) of rice vinegar and mix with 2 cups (500 milliliters) of water. Soak your feet in this mixture for one hour twice every day.
- Boil 1 cup (200 grams) of soybeans in 4 cups (1 liter) of water for 30 minutes. Allow the water to cool and use it wash your feet once a day for two weeks. Prepare fresh every two or three days.

According to Chinese medical theory, athlete's foot is not dependent solely on the damp, humid environment of the foot, but also on a person's physical health and resistance. During the Tang dynasty athlete's foot was observed to be a precursor of beriberi, a disease brought on by a vitamin B_1 deficiency. Therefore, food that is rich in vitamin B_1 is prescribed to combat both athlete's foot and beriberi. Almonds, soybeans, betel nuts, and plantain seed are some of the oldest remedies suggested by the famous long-lived physician Sun Si Miao (A.D. 581–682). Others remedies follow.

Peanuts, Adzuki Beans, and Jujube Decoction

½ cup (100 grams) adzuki beans
Water for soaking
4 cups (1 liter) water
½ cup (100 grams) jujube
½ head (approximately 50 grams) garlic, peeled and lightly
   crushed
⅔ cup (130 grams) raw peanuts, shelled

Soak the adzuki beans in water for at least 2 hours, then drain.

Bring 4 cups of water to boil in a medium saucepan. Place all the ingredients in the boiling water. When the water returns to a boil, reduce the flame to low. Cover. Decoct for 20 minutes over a low flame.

Allow to cool slightly. Drink warm, as part of a meal. The quantity is sufficient for two servings.

Liver and Beans Congee

5 cups (1.25 liters) water
1½ tablespoons (20 grams) mung beans
½ cup (100 grams) pork liver, cut into 1-inch cubes
1 cup (200 grams) rice

In a medium saucepan, bring the water to a boil. Place the beans and the liver in the water, cover the pan, and boil over a low flame for 20 minutes.

Add the rice. Cover the pan again. Cook for 15 minutes, stirring occasionally, to make a congee.

Divide the congee into four portions. Eat one portion, warm, two times a day as part of a meal.

BLOODY STOOLS

Blood in the stools can result from several causes. If the blood is red and fresh, it usually denotes either hemorrhoids or a lesion of the anus or rectum caused by difficult defecation. If the blood is black and dry, the cause of the lesion is usually found further up the alimentary canal. In the latter circumstance, it is best to consult a physician.

The rupture of fragile blood vessels in the anus can be prevented by eating plenty of food rich in soluble fiber. This ensures that the stools are soft and sufficiently bulky.

All of the following remedies ensure the intake of plenty of fiber and are quite straightforward.

- Eat 3 or 4 figs twice a day on an empty stomach. If fresh figs are not in season, dried figs will do.
- Eat 2 bananas every day on an empty stomach.
- Consume 6 to 12 raw pine nuts three times a day.
- Cut 1 cup (200 grams) of radish or daikon into 1/2-inch cubes. Boil in 2 cups (500 milliliters) of water for 15 minutes over a medium flame. Allow to cool, and add honey to taste. Take as a frequent snack.
- Take sunflower seeds frequently as a snack. Sunflower seeds can also be prepared and drunk as a tea.

Sunflower Seed Tea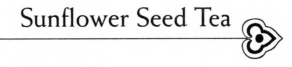

🖐️🖐️🖐️ ✌️

2 tablespoons (30 grams) raw sunflower seeds
2 tablespoons (30 grams) rock sugar
4 cups (1 liter) water

Using a grinding stone or mortar and pestle, grind the sunflower seeds into a powder. Transfer to a cup or bowl, and mix the powder with rock sugar.

In a medium saucepan, combine the powder with the water. Bring to a boil, cover, then reduce heat and simmer over a low flame for 1 hour.

Drink one cup of the tea three times a day, warm.

The following remedies for bloody stools are not based on the intake of a lot of soluble fiber.

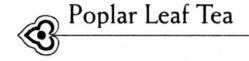# Poplar Leaf Tea

12 fresh poplar leaves
Water for steaming
1 cup water

Wash the poplar leaves and place them in a steaming dish (see page 66). Using a pot deep enough to fit your steamer, bring water to a boil. Put the steamer in the pot, cover, and steam for 10 minutes.

Remove the leaves from the steamer and place them on a flat surface to dry. When they are dry, crumble the leaves.

Boil 1 cup of water. Place 1 teaspoon (5 grams) of the dried poplar leaves in a cup and add boiling water. Cover and steep for at least 5 minutes before drinking.

Drink 1 cup a day.

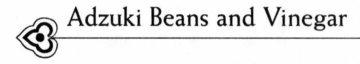# Adzuki Beans and Vinegar

6 cups (1.5 liters) rice vinegar
3 cups (600 grams) adzuki beans

In a medium saucepan, bring the vinegar to a boil. Add the adzuki beans. Simmer over a low flame for 45 minutes, until the vinegar has almost evaporated. Stir frequently.

Transfer the beans to a flat surface and allow them to dry. When dry, grind the beans to a powder with a stone grinder or a mortar and pestle.

Take 1 teaspoon of the powder every morning before breakfast.

BURNS AND SCALDS

Immediate first aid treatment for dry burns should always be to apply cool water to the burn. Cooling is necessary because burned tissues continue to retain heat after the immediate cause of the injury has been removed. This heat can damage deeper layers of skin even several hours after the event.

It is best to plunge the burned area into a basin of cool—not cold—water. (Cold water causes the skin to blister, and the cold-water plunge is painful.) Thrusting the burned area under a running faucet is sufficient if a basin is not available, although strong pressure from the tap might rupture the burned skin. (Or you might, in your panic, turn on the hot tap by mistake!) If the burn is on a part of the body less accessible to a basin plunge, try pouring the water slowly from a pitcher onto the area.

Keep the burn under water for at least ten minutes. After that, what you should do depends on the degree and size of the burn. First-degree burns, and second-degree burns that cover an area one inch in diameter or less, can be treated at home.* Anything more serious must be attended to at a first aid clinic or a hospital. In either case, keep the burn free of clothing or bandages—one school of thought claims that first- and second-degree burns should be treated only with air, oxygen being necessary to the process of tissue regeneration. Chinese medicine holds that, while permitting a burn to "breathe" is necessary, healing will take place more easily by applying various natural products.

If you have developed blisters from a burn, do not burst them. To do so would leave scar tissue and open the underlying raw flesh to possible infections.

The following are common Chinese household remedies for burns.

❖ Soak the burn in a bowl of cool milk, or soak a cotton cloth in milk and apply to the burn.
❖ Crush a carrot and apply to the injured part.
❖ Apply natural honey to the burn. Honey has a cleansing and antibacterial effect.
❖ Fresh ginger juice applied to a burn by means of cotton wool is reported to stop pain instantly, and to reduce inflammation and swelling.
❖ Place slices of fresh cucumber on the skin. This remedy is commonly used for sunburn.
❖ Apply cucumber juice to scalds. Scalds are the most common type of burn sustained in the home, especially those caused by hot tap water.
❖ Place cool slices of raw potato gently against the burn.

* First-degree burns are characterized by redness of the skin—sunburn is a typical example. Second-degree burns are characterized by redness and blistering. Third-degree burns destroy all the skin and some of the underlying muscle and appear dry, leathery, and charred.

- Although yogurt is new to China, it was quickly realized by Chinese people that yogurt applied to first-degree burns, including sunburn, helps to alleviate the discomfort and hasten tissue recovery.[8]
- Aloe vera was introduced to China from central America, and is not, therefore, a traditional remedy. Aloe vera is used in China, as throughout the rest of the world, as a cooling balm for burns. Use either the moist flesh of a cut leaf, or the juice. Apply immediately to first-degree burns, or after the blisters have formed to second- and third-degree burns.

Other remedies are used in China to help the skin heal after emergency treatments have had time to work. Some of these are:

- Place slices of a mature pumpkin inside a jar and bury it in the ground. Leave it for several days, giving the flesh time to rot and liquefy. Then apply the juice to the burn. The application of rotting pumpkin serves to hasten tissue healing several days after the event.
- Mash 2 cakes of tofu, mix with sugar, and apply to the burn.
- Dry some watermelon rind and grind it into a powder. Mix 2 tablespoons (30 grams) of this powder with 1 tablespoon (15 milliliters) of sesame oil, and apply to the burned skin area.
- Blend the white of 1 egg and 1 tablespoon (15 milliliters) of sesame oil. Apply twice a day to the burn.

A diet rich in vitamin C, protein, and liquids is important for recovering from second- and third-degree burns. Raw fruit, especially that which is rich in vitamin C—oranges, kiwi, strawberries—should be eaten in abundance. One should increase one's intake of calories, and especially of protein. Eat tofu, meat, dairy products, and fish. Plenty of liquids should be consumed.

COMMON COLD

According to Chinese theory, there exist two kinds of cold: *feng-han* (wind and cold) and *feng-re* (wind and heat).

Feng-han colds are common in winter and spring. Symptoms are a runny nose, sneezing, liquid catarrh, and no sweating. A feng-re cold, on the other hand, causes a blocked nose that does not run, sore throat, thick and yellow catarrh, thirst, and sweating.

The remedies for feng-han colds are warm diaphoretics (sweat inducers). Those for feng-re colds are diaphoretics with cooling or cold characteristics.

What one eats is particularly important to the progress of the cold. Plenty of hot water should be drunk throughout the day. Eat only food that is light and easily digestible. Liquid foods such as milk, congee, soups, and broths should form the basis of your diet. Refrain from fish, meat, and fats—do not eat lamb, beef, pork, or chicken after taking a diaphoretic to induce sweat. Eat plenty of fruit, especially oranges, kiwis, tomatoes, apples, and pears. Consume green vegetables and salads. Spicy ingredients should not be taken until after the symptoms of the cold have disappeared.

Garlic Nose Drops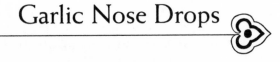

During the initial stages of a cold, when one starts sneezing and the nose begins to run, the first remedy that most Chinese people resort to is garlic drops.

2 fresh garlic cloves, peeled
¹/₄ cup (60 milliliters) water at room temperature

Press the garlic cloves to extract the juice. Mix the garlic juice with water—the proportion should be 1 part garlic juice to 10 parts water.
    Apply the juice as nose drops.

Daikon Nose Drops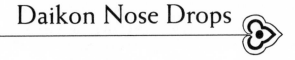

Instead of garlic, which some people find too powerful, you can instead use daikon juice.

1 tablespoon (15 grams) fresh daikon, grated
¹/₄ cup (60 milliliters) water at room temperature

Squeeze the daikon to extract the juice. Mix the juice with water—the proportion should be 1 part daikon juice to 10 parts water.
    Apply the juice as nose drops.

Garlic Pacifier

As well as combating a runny nose, garlic can also be taken orally to prevent a cough and sore throat.

3 garlic cloves

Peel the garlic. Put 1 clove, whole, into your mouth. Leave it there until you can no longer taste it—this can be as long as one hour. Swallow your saliva as it forms. Do not suck with force or chew.

Spit the clove out when it has lost all flavor. When you are ready, start again with a second clove. Later, take the third.

Do this once a day until you feel better.

Ginger and Scallion Soup

A good sweat-inducing recipe for when you feel a cold developing is a hot soup.

2 cups (500 milliliters) water
2 tablespoons (30 grams) fresh ginger, sliced
2 tablespoons (30 grams) white head of scallion, sliced

In a medium saucepan, bring the water to a boil. Add the ginger and scallion and simmer over a low flame for 15 minutes, or until the ginger is soft and its smell has spread through your kitchen.

Drink hot before betime. Stay away from the cold, and especially from cold drafts (the "evil air").

Garlic and Scallion Congee

👍 ✂

The following warming remedy for curing a cold in its early stages is especially effective when the cold is accompanied by a headache.

3 cups (750 milliliters) water
½ cup (100 grams) white rice
3 garlic cloves, finely minced
2 teaspoons (10 grams) minced scallion, white heads only

In a medium saucepan, bring the water to a boil. Add the rice, return to a boil, then lower the flame and simmer for 20 minutes, covered, stirring occasionally.

When the rice has been cooked down to a gruel, add the garlic and scallion. Cook for 5 more minutes over a low flame.

Consume hot once a day, as part of a meal. Wear heavy clothing or get into bed so as to maintain the heat of the congee within your body.

Dandelion and Chrysanthemum Tea

👍👍👍 ✂

1 tablepoon (15 grams) dry dandelion leaves
2 teaspoons (10 grams) dried chrysanthemum flower
2 teaspoons (10 grams) green tea leaves
1 cup (250 milliliters) water

Mix the dandelion leaves, chrysanthemum flower, and tea leaves. Store in a glass jar.

Bring water to a boil. Put 1 heaped teaspoon (5+ grams) of mixed leaves and flowers in a cup. Pour hot water in the cup. Cover and steep for 5 minutes.

Drink hot two times a day.

The following remedies are diaphoretics for feng-han colds (colds characterized by liquid catarrh and a runny nose). These remedies should be taken just before going to bed either at night or, if the cold is bad enough, during the day. Most of these sweat-inducing dishes are based on ginger and the white head of spring onion, or scallion, two of the best diaphoretics available.

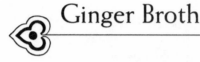

Ginger Broth

In this remedy, the ginger induces sweating and brown sugar promotes circulation.

2 cups (500 milliliters) water
2 tablespoons (30 grams) sliced fresh ginger
Brown sugar to taste

In a small saucepan, bring the water to a boil. Add the ginger. When half the water has evaporated, add the sugar. Continue boiling for 3 minutes.

Take the decoction hot. When you have finished, get under a quilt or blanket for a sweat.

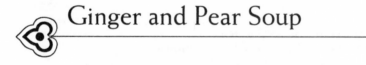

Ginger and Pear Soup

2 cups (500 milliliters) water
1 pear
1 tablespoon (15 grams) sliced fresh ginger
1 tablespoon (15 grams) sliced scallion, white heads only
2 eggs, beaten

Bring the water to a boil in a small saucepan. Cut the pear in half; do not peel it. Add the pear, ginger, and scallion to the water. Return to a boil, cover the pan, and reduce the flame to low. Simmer for 20 minutes.

In the meantime, thoroughly beat the eggs in a glass or ceramic bowl. When the broth is ready—you will know it is when the aroma of ginger spreads through your kitchen—pour the decoction into the bowl containing the two beaten eggs. Mix and drink the decoction while it is still hot, then get under a heavy quilt or thick blanket for a good sweat.

Take this remedy once a day for three or four days, or until the cold goes away.

Ginger and Onion Rice

1 teaspoon (5 grams) sliced fresh ginger
1 scallion, including roots and green tops
1 cup (200 grams) rice
6 cups (1.5 liters) water
2 teaspoons (10 milliliters) rice vinegar

Put the ginger, scallion, rice, and water in a medium saucepan. Bring to a boil, then reduce the flame. Simmer on a low flame with the lid half-covering the saucepan, stirring occasionally. Cook for 25 minutes, or until the rice has becomes a gruel.

Stir in the vinegar. Cook for another minute or two.

Divide into four portions. Take one portion, hot, then get into bed or cover up under a warm blanket. Take this remedy two times a day, while the cold persists.

Egg and Sugar

1 fresh egg
2 tablespoons (30 grams) sugar
1 cup (250 milliliters) water

Beat the egg and sugar together in a bowl.

Bring the water to a boil in a small saucepan. Pour the boiling water over the egg and sugar.

Take hot just before retiring to bed for a good, toxin-flushing sweat.

The following remedies contain cooling ingredients, such as green tea leaves, that balance the sweat-inducing effects of the diaphoretics. These recipes work best for feng-re colds—those with blocked nose, thick catarrh, and cough—which are often accompanied by a headache.

Ginger and Scallion Tea

This remedy is particularly useful for clearing headaches caused by colds.

1½ cups (375 milliliters) water
1 tablespoon (15 grams) sliced fresh ginger
1 tablespoon (15 grams) chopped scallion, white heads only
2 teaspoons (10 grams) green tea leaves

Bring the water to a boil in a small saucepan. Add all the ingredients and boil over a medium flame for 10 minutes.

Drink hot, and stay away from "evil air" (cold and drafts).

(If you are suffering from a fever in addition to a cold, you should add 1 tablespoon (15 grams) of walnut meats to this recipe. Boil for 15 minutes instead of 10.)

Ginger Tea

This effective, fast-acting remedy is good for combating colds that are accompanied by a strong headache.

1 cup (250 milliliters) water
¼ cup (50 grams) fresh ginger, thinly sliced
¼ cup (50 grams) brown sugar
1 teaspoon (5 grams) green tea leaves

Bring the water to a boil in a small saucepan. Add the ginger and sugar. Turn the burner off and wait for 1 minute, then add the tea leaves. (Green tea contains vitamin C; the 1-minute wait after boiling ensures that the vitamin is not destroyed by the heat.) Steep for 5 minutes before drinking.

A frequent addition to this tea is ½ teaspoon (2.5 milliliters) of vinegar. Vinegar exerts a warming and detoxifying effect.

It is recommended that you eat some rice congee immediately after taking this tea.

Sweetened Ginger and Scallion Broth

👍👍👍 ✌️

This remedy is useful when one is soaked to the skin by a sudden rain shower or by falling into water. It is also effective for curing abdominal pains due to catching cold. This broth should be taken just before going to bed.

1 cup (250 milliliters) water
¼ cup (50 grams) fresh ginger, thinly sliced
5 white heads of scallion, thinly sliced
2 teaspoons (20 grams) brown sugar, or more to taste

In a small saucepan, bring the water to a boil. Place the ginger, scallion, and sugar in a cup or bowl. Pour the boiled water over the ingredients. Steep for 5 minutes, then drink.

Retire to a warm bed. The sweat thus induced should leave you feeling better by morning.

Peppermint and Scallion Broth

👍👍👍 ✌️

Peppermint rises to the head (Yang) and has a cooling, pungent effect. It is therefore a good relief for colds accompanied by headaches.

20–30 fresh peppermint leaves, or 2 heaped teaspoons (10+ grams) dried peppermint
2 or 3 crushed white heads of scallion
2 cups (500 milliliters) water

Place all ingredients in a small saucepan. Bring to a boil, then reduce the flame. Simmer for 15 minutes, or until half the water has evaporated.

Drink hot or warm.

Scallion Inhalers

This remedy effectively relieves a blocked nose, it may be used as a natural alternative to vaporubs. In China, this remedy is usually preferred to any over-the-counter medications.

1 white head of scallion, sliced lengthwise

Place the scallion slices directly under your nostrils. Inhale deeply. Continue breathing deeply until your nasal passages are freed.

Watermelon and Tomato Juice

One recipe commonly employed in summer for a hot and dry cold uses watermelon and tomato. Besides curing hot, dry colds, watermelon and tomato combat dehydration, quench thirst, and relieve indigestion and lack of appetite.

2 pounds (1 kilogram) fresh watermelon
2 pounds (1 kilogram) fresh tomatoes

Chop the watermelon and tomatoes into small pieces, keeping them separate. Put them separately into thin cotton towels. Twist each to extract the liquid.

Mix the juices in equal portions. Drink at room temperature, slightly cooled but not cold, as often as you like.

COUGHS

To provide relief for coughs, ginger and onion combinations are prepared with daikon, which has cool, pungent, and sweet characteristics and eliminates hot irritation of the throat and bronchi.

Daikon, Ginger, and Scallion Soup

This popular remedy for coughs and colds also clears catarrh and counteracts body pains, weakness, and lethargy due to colds.

3 cups (750 milliliters) water
1 medium daikon, cut it into ¹/₂-inch slices
1 tablespoon (15 grams) sliced fresh ginger
6 white heads of scallion, sliced

Bring the water to a boil in a medium saucepan. Add the daikon to the water. Continue to boil over a medium flame for 20 minutes, or until the daikon is soft. ("Soft" is defined in China as yielding enough to push the point of a chopstick through the daikon slice with ease).

Add the sliced scallion and ginger to the pot. Reduce the flame to low. Simmer for another 10 minutes, or until two-thirds of the water has evaporated.

Remove from heat. Consume hot.

Daikon and Tangerine Peel Soup

This is a classic remedy for a thick-mucous cough.

1 cup (250 milliliters) water
1 small daikon, cut it into ¹/₂-inch slices
1 organic tangerine peel, cut it into ¹/₂-inch slices
3 slices ginger
1 teaspoon (5 grams) white pepper

In a small saucepan, bring the water to a boil. Add the daikon, tangerine peel, ginger, and pepper to the boiling water. Continue to boil over a medium flame for 10 minutes.

Pour into a bowl and allow to cool. Take the soup twice a day, after lunch and dinner.

Daikon juice on its own is a good remedy for a cold with headache and cough, as well as for chronic bronchitis. If the cough is particularly persistent, daikon juice can be mixed with ginger and pear juice and the white of an egg.

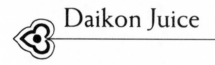

Daikon Juice

4 cups (800 grams) fresh daikon, grated
1 tablespoon (15 grams) brown sugar

Place the daikon in a thin cotton towel and squeeze in order to obtain the juice. Mix the juice and brown sugar in a small saucepan. Bring to a boil over medium heat.

Remove from the flame and allow to cool. Drink the juice two times a day, warm to hot, to relieve coughing.

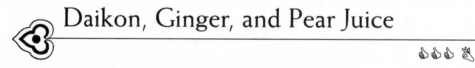

Daikon, Ginger, and Pear Juice

½ cup (100 grams) fresh daikon, grated
½ cup (100 grams) fresh ginger, grated
2 tablespoons (30 milliliters) fresh pear juice
1 egg white

Place the daikon in a thin cotton towel and squeeze to extract 2 tablespoons of juice. Repeat with the ginger.

Mix the ginger and daikon juice with the pear juice and egg white. Drink it cool once a day.

Daikon Juice Drops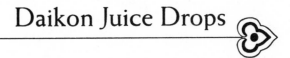

👍👍👍 ✋

½ cup (100 grams) fresh daikon, grated

Place the daikon in a thin cotton towel and squeeze in order to obtain the juice. Use the juice directly as nose drops.

Garlic is another popular remedy for persistent coughs.

Garlic Juice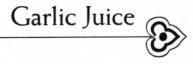

👍👍👍 ✋

1–2 cups (200–400 grams) fresh garlic cloves
1 cup (250 milliliters) water
1 teaspoon (5 grams) white sugar

Peel and squeeze the garlic in order to extract the juice. Transfer to a clean bottle or jar and refrigerate.

When you need to use a cough remedy, boil 1 cup of water. Mix 1 tablespoon (15 milliliters) of garlic juice and the sugar into the hot water.

To be taken twice a day, morning and evening, until the cough has cleared. Drink the mixture hot.

Garlic Cough Powder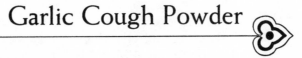

👍👍👍 ✋

1 tablespoon (15 grams) garlic powder
1 teaspoon (5 grams) sugar, white or brown

Mix the garlic powder with the sugar. Take the mixed powder twice daily, with lunch and dinner.

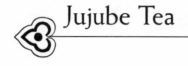

Jujube Tea

A favorite remedy for coughs is the jujube (Chinese date).

5 jujube (Chinese dates)
1 tablespoon (15 grams) minced fresh ginger
1 tablespoon (15 grams) brown sugar
2 cups (500 milliliters) water

In a small saucepan, add all the dry ingredients to the water. Boil over a low flame for 15 minutes.
Consume warm.

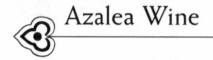

Azalea Wine

¹/₂ cup (100 grams) azalea flowers
4 cups (1 liter) rice wine, or sake

Wash the azalea flowers. Allow them to dry in the shade.
When the flowers are dry, finely chop them. Place the rice wine and the flowers inside a bottle. Seal the bottle. Allow the mixture to macerate for at least 5 days.
Take 2 or 3 teaspoons (10 or 15 milliliters) two times a day.

Other ingredients for cough mixtures include celery, tofu, and lard. Drink one glass of fresh celery juice twice a day, morning and evening, for as long as the cough persists. Tofu and ginger are an effective remedy for chronic coughs, especially those due to chronic bronchitis. And while the final recipe for treating coughs may seem unusual, honey and lard have been used in China for centuries to relieve dry coughs without catarrh.

Tofu and Ginger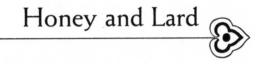

👍👍👍 👌

3 cups (750 milliliters) water
8 ounces (200 grams) tofu, cut into 1-inch cubes
6 tablespoons (90 grams) brown sugar
2 teaspoons (10 grams) crushed ginger

In a medium saucepan, bring the water to a boil. Add all ingredients to the water. Boil over a medium flame for 15 minutes.

Remove the pan from the heat. Consume warm as a gruel once a day, before bed.

Honey and Lard

👍👍👍 👌

This recipe serves an additional purpose: that of ensuring regular bowel movements.

8 tablespoons (120 grams) lard
8 tablespoons (120 grams) honey

In a small saucepan, heat the ingredients over a low flame, bringing them to a boil. Remove from heat and allow to cool.

Consume when the mixture cools sufficiently to become creamy and opaque.

CONSTIPATION

For optimum health the bowels should be cleared daily. Fecal matter that stays in the intestines for longer than twenty-four hours causes harmful bacteria to spread through the system. Furthermore, chronic constipation can lead to abdominal pain, diverticulitis, hemorrhoids, headaches, insomnia, digestive problems, obesity, circulatory problems, hernia, and cancer of the bowel.

A diet of fresh, raw, leafy green vegetables, fresh fruits, and plenty of fiber helps to produce easy bowel movements. Plenty of water (drunk hot in China) or pure fruit juice is needed to dissolve the added intake of fiber. One may resort to natural laxatives; a few are mentioned below. These have been used for centuries in China. Chemical products should not be used—they are too thorough in cleaning out the intestines, killing all bacteria and giving rise to chronic constipation.

To prevent constipation it is important to exercise. Any exercise will do because all physical activity helps move waste matter through the intestines. Qi gong breathing exercises are especially beneficial in that they exert a salutary, massaging effect on the abdominal and intestinal areas, thus facilitating the elimination of fecal matter.

In a variation of the qi gong standing position that has been designed specifically to relieve constipation, stand with your back straight and knees slightly bent (see page 245). Place your hands on your hips and rotate your pelvis to the left, then to the front, then right, and then back for five to ten minutes each the morning.

Before proceeding with the remedies here, a few words may be in order about Chinese toilet habits. It is believed that people defecate best if they concentrate. Do not therefore take a book or other distraction to the toilet with you—concentrate solely on the matter at hand. Push and, as Chinese parents tell their children, clench your teeth.

In the course of our research, we discovered numerous easy home remedies for the common ailment of constipation. We leave the choice of remedy to the reader.

- Simply add salt to warm water and drink. The more salt you add, the more powerful the effect. Take care: you may find yourself throwing up as well.
- Add 1 tablespoon (15 milliliters) of vinegar to a large glass of warm or hot water. Drink in the morning on an empty stomach. Follow this by another glass of warm or hot water without the vinegar. Go out for a thirty- to sixty-minute walk. On your return, repair to the bathroom.

Some foods taken regularly as part of one's diet are known to facilitate easy and daily bowel movements.

- One of the gentlest and yet most efficient ways of ensuring regular bowel movements is to eat leafy green vegetables.
- Nearly as effective as eating the vegetables is drinking their juice—all leafy green vegetables will work. Extract the juice of the green leaf vegetable of your choice, or boil in water and drink the broth.
- Take 2 soft, very ripe bananas every morning and evening.
- Roast 2 tablespoons (30 grams) of black sesame seeds in a dry frying pan for 3 minutes. Eat the sesame with 1 or 2 ripe bananas. This remedy counteracts both constipation and high blood pressure.

❖ Take 2 teaspoons (10 milliliters) of honey twice a day, morning and evening. Continue for two weeks. You may mix the honey with warm water and drink.

❖ Stir 1 teaspoon (5 milliliters) of honey and ¹/₂ teaspoon (2.5 milliliters) of sesame oil in a glass of hot water. Take before going to bed.

❖ Steam 2 cups (400 grams) of honey and 2 cups (400 grams) of lard together in a large ceramic bowl for 15 minutes (see page 66). Store in a jar. Take 1 tablespoon every morning and evening on an empty stomach. This recipe is also used for treating dry coughs with little catarrh.

❖ Wash 1 cup (200 grams) of figs. Boil the figs in 4 cups (1 liter) of water over a low flame for 20 minutes. Drink the juice as a tea, with a little sugar added according to taste.

❖ Drink the white of 1 raw egg every morning with your breakfast. You may mix with fruit juice or any other cool drink. Grapefruit is said to be the best fruit juice remedy for constipation.

❖ Drink a glass of fresh grapefruit every day before breakfast, on an empty stomach.

Honey and Potato Juice

2 pounds (1 kilogram) potatoes, washed but not peeled
1 tablespoon (15 milliliters) honey

Cut the potatoes into ¹/₂-inch cubes. Using a thin cotton towel, squeeze the potatoes over a small saucepan to extract the juice.

Heat the juice on a high flame; lower the flame as the juice begins to boil. Add honey and simmer for 5 to 10 minutes until creamy.

Remove from flame. Let cool, then store in a jar or bottle and refrigerate.

Take 1 tablespoon (15 milliliters) once a day, in the morning before breakfast. If you forget you can take it anytime, but always do so on an empty stomach. (In another version of this recipe, the honey and potato juice are mixed cold and drunk raw.)

Sesame, Walnut, and Pine Kernel Muesli

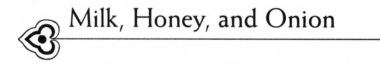

2 tablespoons (30 grams) sesame seeds, black or white
2 tablespoons (30 grams) walnut meats
2 tablespoons (30 grams) pine nuts
2 tablespoons (30 grams) honey

Chop and then grind the sesame, walnuts, and pine nuts, using a stone grinder or a mortar and pestle. Work the ingredients into granules, then add the honey and mix into a paste.

Consume every morning with your breakfast.

Milk, Honey, and Onion

½ cup (100 grams) white onion, chopped fine
1 cup (250 milliliters) milk
8 tablespoons (90 grams) honey

Using a thin cotton towel, squeeze the onion for its juice.

In a small saucepan, bring the milk to a boil. Add the onion juice and allow to simmer for 1 minute. Remove from the flame.

Allow to cool for 5 minutes. Stir in the honey.

Drink warm every morning on an empty stomach.

Onion Compress

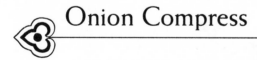

This onion remedy is especially effective for women suffering from constipation after childbirth. It serves to stimulate bowel movement by exerting a warming and relaxing effect on the outside of the abdomen.

Hot water
½ cup (100 grams) onion, finely chopped

Place a towel in hot water. When it is soaked through, remove the towel from the wash basin and squeeze out the excess moisture. Lie down on your back and apply the onion to your navel. Place the hot towel over the onion. Hold the towel in place for 5 minutes.

Reheat the towel and repeat for another 5 minutes. You can, if you prefer, use a hot water bottle instead of a towel. In the latter case, hold in place for 10 minutes.

Onion, Ginger, and Radish Juice Compress

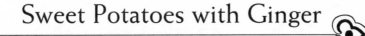

    ¹/₂ cup (100 grams) daikon, grated
    1 tablespoon (15 grams) onion, chopped
    1 teaspoon (5 grams) ginger, chopped
    4 teaspoons (20 grams) salt

Squeeze the daikon to extract 1 tablespoon of juice into a glass.

In a wok or frying pan, stir-fry the onion, ginger, salt, and daikon juice together for 3 minutes.

Remove from the heat and allow to cool. Wrap the mixture in a thin cloth and apply to your navel once a day until you feel well again. Keep the compress in place for 20 minutes.

Sweet Potatoes with Ginger

    4 cups (1 liter) water
    1 sweet potato, cut in ¹/₂-inch slices
    1 4-ounce (100-gram) piece of ginger, cut in ¹/₂-inch slices
    2 tablespoons (30 grams) sugar, white or brown

In a medium saucepan, bring the water to a boil. Add the sweet potato, ginger, and sugar. Boil over a medium flame for 15–20 minutes, until the sweet potato is edible.

Remove from the flame. Mash and consume as part of a meal.

This dish may be eaten as frequently as you like.

Steamed Eggplant

1 eggplant (aubergine), peeled and cut in ¼-inch slices
Water for steaming
Salt or oil to taste

Place the eggplant in a ceramic bowl or steaming dish (see page 66). Using a pot deep enough to fit your steamer, bring water to a boil. Put the steamer in the pot, cover, and steam for 10 minutes.

Eat warm once a day, as often as you like. Add salt or oil if you wish.

Cooked Spinach

1 cup (200 grams) fresh packed spinach
2 tablespoons (30 milliliters) water
1 teaspoon (5 milliliters) sesame oil

Place the spinach in a wok or medium saucepan with the water. Setting the flame on high, stir the spinach for 2 minutes.

Remove from the flame and allow to cool. Add sesame oil. Eat warm.

Sesame Eggs

In China, black sesame seed is considered to be an effective laxative. Sesame can be eaten with eggs, or with rice as a congee.

½ cup (100 grams) black sesame seeds
1 teaspoon (5 grams) salt
1 egg
1 cup (250 milliliters) water

Roast the sesame seeds in a dry frying pan or wok over a low flame for 3 minutes, or until you can smell the distinct odor of sesame. Add salt, and roast for another 30 seconds.

Place the egg in a small saucepan with the water. Bring to a boil, then boil for 10 minutes.

Allow the egg to cool, then cut into segments. Mix the egg with the sesame. Consume warm, two times a day.

Black Sesame Congee

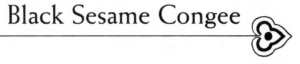

¹/₂ cup (100 grams) white rice
3 cups (750 milliliters) water
2 tablespoons (30 grams) black sesame seeds

In a medium saucepan, bring the water to a boil. Add the rice and boil over a low flame for 20 minutes.

Crush the sesame seeds with mortar and pestle or stone grinder. Add the sesame to the congee. Simmer for 10 additional minutes.

Take with meals.

Pine nuts or watermelon seeds may be used in this dish as an alternative to sesame:

❖ Prepare a rice congee (see page 69). Roast 2 tablespoons (30 grams) of pine nuts in a dry wok or frying pan for 3 minutes. Crush the pine nuts and add to the congee.

❖ Prepare a congee (see page 69). Roast 2 tablespoons (30 grams) watermelon seeds in a dry wok or frying pan for 4 minutes. Crush the watermelon seeds and add to the congee.

Sometimes even the best laxatives cannot dislodge stubborn constipation. Before resorting to an enema, you might wish to try something of immediate efficacy. This remedy is as straightforward as it is effective.

Take the white head of one scallion; wash and remove the roots. Cover the scallion it with 1 teaspoon of honey. Squat or lie down and slide the scallion up your anus. Keep it in place for 3 minutes.

CORNS

Remedies for corns—the hardening of the skin on the toes—were offered by many people. The following are some of the least complicated to apply.

❖ Squeeze the juice from an eggplant and apply to the corn two or three times a day.

❖ Crush an unripe fig and apply to the corn. Hold in place with a bandage. Change the application twice a day. Seven to ten days of treatment should eliminate the corn.

❖ Apply the white sap of a freshly picked fig directly onto the corn.

❖ Peel the soft transparent skin from a scallion. Before going to bed, wash your foot in hot water and dry. Apply the scallion skin to the corn. Rub gently. Hold in place overnight with either a cloth bandage or Band-Aid. Repeat every evening until the corn becomes soft and white and eventually falls away of its own accord.

Some Chinese chiropodists (foot doctors) assert that the corn should be filed or cut down before making the application. Others argue that no manual intervention is necessary—indeed, that filing or cutting the corn can irritate the surrounding area and can therefore be harmful.

The last remedy for corns is a little more elaborate and will thus need a few minutes of preparation.

Garlic and Onion

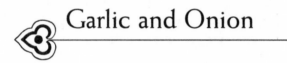

1 head of garlic, minced
1 purple onion, diced
1 teaspoon (5 milliliters) vinegar
8 cups (2 liters) water
1 teaspoon (5 grams) salt

In a small bowl, mix the garlic and onion with the vinegar.

Warm the water in a large saucepan. Add the salt to the water. Cut away the thick skin from the corn. Soak the foot in the warm salty water for about 20 minutes, until the skin is soft. Dry the area around the corn.

Apply 1 tablespoon of the chopped onion and garlic to the corn and rub in well. Cover with a bandage. Apply every four hours, if possible. Store the unused garlic and onion mixture in the refrigerator.

Repeat each day for 5 to 7 days. The fresher the onion and garlic, the more effective the remedy.

DIARRHEA

Diarrhea is a symptom with many possible causes. According to Chinese medicine, the causes can range from a weak spleen and stomach to indigestion, overeating, or cold. The patient usually suffers from abdominal pains, has no appetite, feels lethargic, and needs to run to the toilet many times a day. When things get worse, it is probably not diarrhea but dysentery—see pages 135–138 for more powerful remedies.

In China, garlic is considered to be nature's most effective stomach and intestinal disinfectant. Many people won't travel without it, chewing a clove or two whenever in doubt about local conditions of cleanliness. Garlic's proven antibiotic effects render it a valid remedy for diarrhea.

Garlic and Sugar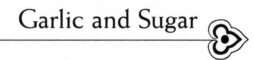

👍👍👍 ✌

3 garlic cloves, peeled
2 teaspoons (20 grams) brown sugar
Water for steaming

Put the garlic cloves in a small ceramic bowl, then put the bowl inside a steaming dish (see page 66). Using a pan deep enough to hold your steamer, bring the water to a boil. Place the steamer in the pan, cover, and steam for 10 minutes.

When the garlic is done, crush it, mix with the sugar, and eat.

Alternatively, you can crush the raw garlic, then boil it in 1 cup (250 milliliters) of water with sugar.

Taken two or three times a day, these are both effective remedies for chronic diarrhea and intestinal gases.

Garlic Broth

👍👍👍 ✌

2 or 3 garlic cloves, unpeeled
1 cup (250 milliliters) water

Roast the garlic in a small, dry saucepan until the skin begins to darken. Add the water. Bring to a boil over a medium flame; continue to boil for 5 minutes.

Remove from heat. Drink warm.

119

Garlic and Eggs

Garlic taken with eggs is doubly efficacious in that it counteracts diarrhea accompanied by general weakness.

3 garlic cloves, peeled
2 eggs
1 teaspoon (5 milliliters) sesame oil

Squeeze the juice from the garlic. In a small bowl, beat the garlic juice with the raw eggs.

Heat the sesame oil in a wok or frying pan. When the oil is hot, pour in the eggs and garlic and stir-fry for 1 to 2 minutes.

To be taken twice a day.

Garlic Vinegar

The following remedy is recommended primarily for diarrhea; it is, however, also effective for treating gastroenteritis. It can be taken as a preventive measure, as well as for curing both diarrhea and gastroenteritis.

4 garlic cloves, minced
3 tablespoons (45 milliliters) vinegar

Squeeze the garlic into a glass to extract the juice. Add vinegar. Sip slowly.

Garlic vinegar may also be prepared by maturing 18 cloves of garlic in 3 cups (750 milliliters) of vinegar for 24 hours. Take 6 cloves for breakfast, 6 for lunch, and 6 for dinner. Repeat each day until cured.

Ginger Tea

👍👍👍 ✌️

2 teaspoons (10 grams) green tea leaves
2 teaspoons (10 grams) minced ginger
2 cups (500 milliliters) water

Prepare a decoction by boiling the tea leaves, ginger, and water over a low flame, covered, for 20 minutes.
    Drink the decoction hot.

Ginger and Scallion Omelet

👍👍 ✌️

3 eggs
1 tablespoon (15 grams) finely chopped ginger
1 scallion, finely chopped
1 tablespoon (15 milliliters) rice vinegar
Salt to taste

In a small bowl, beat the eggs with the chopped ginger and scallion.
    Pour the rice vinegar into a medium frying pan. Heat, then add the eggs, ginger, and scallion mixture.
    Cook over a high flame for 3 minutes. Using a spatula, turn the omelette and cook the front side for 1 minute.
    Remove from heat and slide the omelette from the pan. Eat once a day until you feel better.

Boiled Apples

👍👍👍 ✌️

10 green apples
16 cups (4 liters) water

In a large pot, bring the water to a boil. Add the apples and boil them whole over a low flame for 40 minutes, until soft.
    Eat as many as you can on an empty stomach.

Chestnut Cakes

Chestnut strengthens zheng qi, the intestines, and the stomach. It also exerts a strong warming and curative effect on cold-syndrome diarrhea.

¹/₄ cup (50 grams) chestnut flour
Sugar to taste
2 tablespoons (30 milliliters) water
Water for steaming

In a small bowl, blend the flour and sugar with water. Divide the dough and roll into four round cakes.

Put the cakes in a steaming dish (see page 66). Using a pan deep enough to fit your steamer, bring water to a boil. Place your steamer inside the pan, cover, and steam for 20 minutes. (If you wish, you may instead bake the cakes at 350°F for 20 minutes.)

Eat the cakes warm. Remember to apply the maxim "Drink your food and eat your drinks." Make sure that each piece of food is well and properly chewed, and is swallowed with plenty of saliva. Chestnut contains starch, and the digestion of starch begins with saliva.

Pork Gall and Honey

A traditional remedy that is used in the Chinese countryside to cure liver problems, as well as diarrhea, is one using pork gallbladder.

1 gallbladder of pork
8 tablespoons (120 milliliters) honey
Water for steaming

Chop the gallbladder into cubes. Place it in a thin cotton towel and squeeze to obtain the gall. Transfer the gall to a bowl. Stir in the honey.

Put the mixture in a ceramic bowl on a steaming dish (see page 66). Using a pan deep enough to fit your steamer, bring water to a boil. Place your steamer inside the pan and cover. Steam for 15 minutes.

Take the whole remedy in one sitting. One dose should clear the problem.

Remedies of the kind that follow, in which ingredients are applied to the skin, may be received with a little superstition. Skin applications are popular in Chinese medicine, and are now becoming increasingly acceptable remedies in mainstream Western medicine. By passing through the pores of the skin directly into the capillaries, it is believed that the ingredients may exert a more immediate, albeit milder, effect than by ingestion.

Garlic and Pepper Compress

👍👍👍 ✌️

2 garlic cloves
8 peppercorns, black or white

Chop the garlic and pepper together to make fine granules. Compress the granules into two cakes.

Bind the cakes to the underside of the feet against the center of the sole, or apply the whole amount to your navel as you lie on your back. Keep in place overnight.

Onion and Salt Compress

👍👍👍 ✌️

This compress is said to work best for diarrhea due to cold syndromes; it also provides effective relief from abdominal pains.

¹/₂ cup (100 grams) onion, chopped
1 tablespoon (15 grams) rock salt

In a dry frying pan or wok, roast the onion together with the salt. When hot, place the salt and onion inside a cotton sachet. Apply as hot as is comfortable to the abdomen, lower back, and waist.

Apply twice each day for as long as the problem lasts.

Other simple food remedies for diarrhea include the following.

♦ Eat 1 peeled crab apple first thing in the morning, before breakfast. Eat more during the day.
♦ Drink 1 cup (250 milliliters) of fresh radish juice on an empty stomach once or twice a day.
♦ Roast 1 whole tuber of ginger in a dry wok or frying pan for 10 minutes, until the outside is dark and dry. Grind the tuber into a powder. Take 1 teaspoon of the powder with warm water three times a day.

DYSENTERY

Dysentery, like food poisoning, is common whenever the climate and poor sanitary conditions encourage bacteria to proliferate, hence the common travelers' complaints of Delhi belly, curse of the pharaohs, and Montezuma's revenge. Symptoms of acute bacillary dysentery are a continuous urgent need to use the toilet; watery stools, sometimes containing blood and puss; nausea; vomiting; abdominal pain; and fever. Chronic amoebic dysentery is slightly less severe in its initial manifestation—there may be no nausea or vomiting—but symptoms persist longer, sometimes for several months. Chronic amoebic dysentery can leave one weak, dehydrated, and many pounds thinner.

The prime defense against bacilli in China is (once again) garlic, the ubiquitous disinfectant of Chinese remedies.

♦ Raw garlic is a strong and effective antibiotic; however, it exerts an irritating effect on the colon. Raw garlic should therefore only be used sparingly in acute cases of dysentery. If the dysentery is chronic you may take garlic raw—2 or 3 cloves at a time—three times a day for one week.
♦ Alternatively, you may crush 1 head of garlic and mix it with 4 teaspoons (20 grams) of sugar. Take three times a day.
♦ Boiled garlic is less irritating to the mucous membranes than raw garlic, and some of its antibiotic effects remain intact. Boiled garlic may therefore be used both for cases of acute and chronic dysentery. Boil a whole garlic head in 1 cup (250 milliliters) of water for 10 minutes, until it is very soft. Remove the skin and mash the flesh with 4 tablespoons (60 grams) of brown sugar. Take twice a day.
♦ Peel 4 or 5 cloves of garlic, then boil them in a small saucepan containing 2 cups (500 milliliters) of water. After 2 minutes of boiling, remove the garlic and add 1/4 cup (50 grams) of rice. Simmer over a low flame for 20 minutes to make a congee, adding water if necessary. When the rice is soft, add the preboiled garlic to the gruel; stir well, then cook for another 3 minutes. To be eaten twice a day for as long as the dysentery persists.

Other food remedies for dysentery include apples, radish, and ginger.

Radish and Ginger Tea

♨ ♨ ♨

> 1 4-ounce (125-gram) piece of ginger, grated
> 16 ounces (500 grams) radish or daikon
> 1 heaping teaspoon (5+ grams) green tea leaves
> 1 cup (250 milliliters) water
> 2 tablespoons (30 milliliters) honey

Over a small bowl, squeeze the grated ginger to extract 1 tablespoon (15 milliliters) of juice. Squeeze the grated radish or daikon over the same bowl to extract 4 tablespoons (70 milliliters) of juice.

Place the tea leaves in a cup. Heat the water in a small saucepan. When the water is about to boil, pour it over the tea leaves. Leave the tea to brew for 10 minutes.

Stir in the ginger and radish juice and honey. Drink warm two or three times a day.

Ginger, Tangerine, and Apple Peel Decoction

♨ ♨ ♨

> 4 teaspoons (20 grams) organic apple peel
> 2 teaspoons (10 grams) organic tangerine peel
> 2 cups (500 milliliters) water
> 1 teaspoon (5 grams) ginger, peeled and sliced

Wash and peel 1 organic apple and 1 organic tangerine.

In a small saucepan, bring the water to a boil. Add the apple, tangerine peel, and ginger slices, and boil over a low flame for 15 minutes.

Drink warm or at room temperature two or three times a day.

Eggs and Ginger

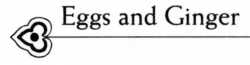

This recipe affects the large intestines and the lungs. It is most effective in allaying a dysentery problem at its onset. Ginger has warming qualities; it induces perspiration and disperses cold. Eggs are sweet and lubricating.

2 eggs
2 teaspoons (10 grams) ginger, finely minced
Water for steaming

Beat the eggs in a small ceramic bowl. Add the ginger to the eggs, then put the bowl in a steaming dish (see page 66).

Using a pan deep enough to fit your steamer, bring water to a boil. Place the steamer in the pan and cover. Steam for 10 minutes.

Take two times a day on an empty stomach.

Green Tea with Vinegar

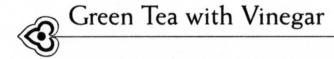

The following concoction is not the best way to enjoy a cup of tea. Quite apart from the vinegar, 100 grams of tea leaves produces a foul, bitter brew. Strong tea, however, is known to detoxify or, in Chinese terms, to relieve internal heat. It is also an efficient diuretic.

1¹/₂ cups (375 milliliters) water
6 tablespoons (90 grams) green tea leaves
6 teaspoons (30 milliliters) vinegar

In a small saucepan, bring the water to a boil. Add the tea leaves and boil over a low flame for 1 minute.

Remove the tea from heat and brew for 5 minutes. Pour equal quantities of tea into three separate cups. Add 2 teaspoons (10 milliliters) of vinegar to each cup.

Drink each cup separately: one in the morning, another in the afternoon, and the third in the evening. Reheat the tea each time to drink it hot.

An alternative to this recipe is to mix the tea with wine instead of vinegar. Although rice wine, or sake, is a less effective than vinegar, it does without a doubt make for a more pleasurable drink.

Tomato Plant Decoction

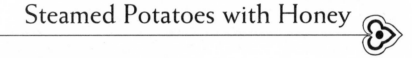

16 cups (4 liters) water
2 or 3 tomato plants, complete with stalks and leaves (no
fruits)

Bring the water to a boil in a large soup kettle. Wash the tomato plants and remove the roots. Cut the plant into 5-inch-long segments. Place the tomato plants in the water and simmer for 3 hours over a low flame.

After boiling, pass the liquid through a strainer. Drink a cup of the decoction every two hours, warm or at room temperature.

Steamed Potatoes with Honey

1 cup (250 milliliters) water
2 or 3 potatoes, peeled and cubed
2 tablespoons (30 milliliters) honey

In a medium saucepan, bring water to a boil.

Place the potatoes in a steaming dish. Put the dish in the saucepan, cover, and steam the potatoes for 15 minutes. When the potatoes are finished steaming, transfer them to a bowl and add honey. Take two or three times a day for as long as the problem persists.

Additional food remedies are as follows:

- Munch an apple well, the greener the apple, the better, or, better still, grate it before you eat it. Eat 3 to 6 apples a day.
- Hard boil 10 to 20 eggs. Eat the yolks until your mouth tastes like *ji shi*. This expression literally translates as "chicken shit," and is, in fact, a genuine Chinese instruction. Do not take this remedy for longer than a week.
- Squeeze 2 or 3 tablespoons (15 or 30 milliliters) of onion juice and mix with the same quantity of vinegar. Bring to a boil in a small saucepan. Remove from the flame; sip hot.

FOOD POISONING

Food poisoning is not a common occurrence in the United States. Nevertheless, mistakes are made: food may become contaminated by toxic bacteria, or one may eat poisonous plants, fish, or mushrooms.

In China, people are fairly careful not to contaminate food. We rarely keep fresh food for more than a few hours. We do not use frozen foods that may go bad during an electricity outage. If we are ever suspicious about sanitary conditions when we travel, we eat our food with plenty of raw garlic because garlic is a natural antibiotic that kills off any harmful bacteria.

Mushroom poisoning is, however, another matter. In China, mushrooms have been used both as food and for medicinal purposes since time immemorial. Only a few species of mushrooms are cultivated; most varieties cannot be grown at will. People therefore pick wild mushrooms at the risk of consuming toxic or poisonous species.

Very few wild mushrooms are deadly, and only one of these has no known antidote. This is the *Amanita phalloides*, or death cap. The reason for this mushroom's extreme toxicity is that it contains three kinds of poison that damage cells throughout the body after being absorbed into the bloodstream. Symptoms of *Amanita phalloides* poisoning therefore appear after digestion is complete, generally between six and fifteen hours after eating. Symptoms include strong abdominal pains, nausea, vomiting, intense thirst, bloody diarrhea, absence of urine, prostration, and convulsions. If any suspicion of *Amanita phalloides* poisoning exists, rush the patient to a hospital that can circulate the patient's blood outside the body through a special charcoal filter, which will eliminate the poison. Nothing else can help.

Other types of mushroom poisoning are less dangerous. Symptoms appear during digestion and can range from stomach pains and nausea to hallucinations. For these forms of mushroom poisoning Chinese peasants have come up with several remedies, all of which are useful in treating all forms of food poisoning.

First of all, one must induce vomiting. To induce vomiting you can drink salt water in large enough quantities to make you vomit, or thrust your fingers down your throat until you retch and throw up.

Once the toxins have been eliminated from the digestive tract, one can administer the following traditional remedies for mushroom poisoning with greater ease.

❖ Grind 1 cup (200 grams) of raw mung beans to a fine powder. Stir 2 tablespoons (30 grams) of powder into 1 cup (250 milliliters) of water. Drink as many cups as you can manage.

❖ Boil ½ cup (100 grams) of soybeans in 4 cups (1 liter) of water over a low flame for 45 minutes. Add water if necessary. Take 1 cup of the soup, warm, twice a day.

❖ Another common antidote to food poisoning is lotus leaf tea. Although common in China, in the United States lotus leaves are available only in specialized Chinese food stores. However, this remedy is worth knowing about in case you need a cure for mushroom poisoning, and lotus leaves are at hand.

   Boil 2 teaspoons (10 grams) of lotus leaves in 2 cups (500 milliliters) of water for 30 minutes, until the brew reduces to 1 cup (250 milliliters). If necessary, add water during the preparation. Drink 1 cup three times a day, until the symptoms of poisoning recede.

❖ Tofu is sometimes poorly prepared, and its ingestion can result in quite severe abdominal pain and nausea. The prescribed remedy for this condition is to drink radish juice. Grate and squeeze enough fresh radishes to extract 1 glass of juice to drink. Alternatively you can boil 12 radishes in 3 cups (750 milliliters) of water for 30 minutes, then drink the soup.

❖ One of the most common forms of food poisoning is that which occurs from eating prawns and shellfish. The Chinese remedy for this is to drink a tea prepared from orange peel. Peel 1 organic orange, then cut the peel into ¹/₂-inch slices. Boil in 1 cup (250 milliliters) of water over a medium flame for 10 to 15 minutes. Drink hot or warm three times a day.

GASTRITIS

Acute gastritis is caused by food poisoning, infection, or excessive eating or drinking. It appears and subsides rapidly. The best cure for gastritis is complete abstinence from food.

   Chronic gastritis, on the other hand, usually depends on the habitual heavy use of irritants such as chili and pepper in one's diet, and on psychosomatic causes such as anxiety, stress, and frustration.

   The obvious solution is to eliminate the irritants and to relax. You might also wish to try one of the following Chinese remedies.

Potato Juice and Honey

👍👍👍 ✌

   1 potato, peeled and grated
   1 teaspoon (5 grams) honey

Using a thin cotton towel, squeeze the potato over a glass to extract the juice. Add honey.

   Drink on an empty stomach every morning for twenty days.

129

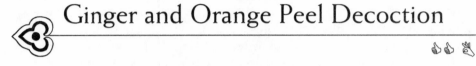

Ginger and Orange Peel Decoction

2 cups (500 milliliters) water
1 tablespoon (15 grams) sliced ginger
1 organic orange peel, sliced

In a small saucepan, bring the water to a boil. Add the ginger and orange peel. Simmer on a low flame for 20 minutes.

Allow the decoction to cool slightly. Drink two or three times a day.

Powdered Eggshell

This classic Chinese remedy checks acidity and gastritis and helps cure duodenal and stomach ulcers.

1 chicken eggshell

In a dry wok or frying pan roast the empty eggshell over a low flame for approximately 4 minutes, or until it is thoroughly dry. Remove and allow the shell to cool, then transfer it to a pestle or stone grinder and grind it into a powder.

Take 1 teaspoon of the powder in warm water before meals.

The same effects are obtained from cuttlefish bone. Bake a cuttlefish and extract the bone, then roast it and grind it into a powder. Take 1 teaspoon (5 grams) of the powder with warm water, again before meals.

Peanuts, Milk, and Honey

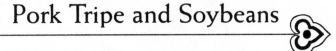

$^1/_4$ **cup (50 grams) raw peanuts**
Water for soaking
1 cup (250 milliliters) milk
2 tablespoons (30 milliliters) honey

Soak the peanuts in hot water for 1 hour. Drain the water, then grind the peanuts to a pulp.

In a small saucepan, bring the milk to a boil. Add the peanuts as soon as the milk begins to rise. Allow the milk to boil again. As the milk rises a second time, remove the saucepan from the flame.

Let cool for 5 minutes. Stir in the honey.

Drink warm just before going to bed.

Pork Tripe and Soybeans

This recipe not only alleviates chronic gastritis, but also helps to recover strength if one has been weakened by gastric problems.

$^1/_2$ **cup (100 grams) soybeans**
Water for soaking
6 cups (1.5 liters) water
8 ounces (250 grams) pork tripe, washed and sliced

Soak the soybeans in 2 cups (500 milliliters) of water overnight. When you are ready to prepare the remedy, drain the soybeans and discard the soaking water.

In a large saucepan, bring 6 cups (1.5 liters) of water to a boil. Add the tripe and boil over a low flame for 1 hour. Add the soybeans to the tripe and continue to boil over a medium flame for another 40 minutes. If necessary, occasionally add small quantities of water.

When done, separate into three equal portions. Consume one portion with each meal: breakfast, lunch, and dinner.

HAIR LOSS AND PREMATURE GRAYING

Hair loss and premature graying may be caused by a wide variety of factors, the most common of which are hereditary. When genes are responsible there is little that one can do about hair problems, except to stay fit and healthy in order to delay as long as possible that which is truly inevitable.

Hair loss and graying that are not hereditary are considered to be due either to weakness in the kidneys and the blood or to poor nourishment of the hair follicles. A poorly balanced diet is said to cause the hair follicles to open and xie qi (evil qi) to enter. The xie qi dries and heats the blood which thus no longer feeds the already undernourished roots, thereby causing the hair to fall out or to lose its color.

Healthy hair depends on good nutrition. Good general health means good healthy hair, and healthy skin for that matter. In China we eat many foods throughout our lives that we consider to be specifically for the health of our hair and skin. Some of these foods are seaweed, sunflower seeds, jujube, apples, plums, scallions, carrots, celery, radish, yogurt, black beans, and peanuts. Walnuts, usually taken first thing in the morning on an empty stomach, are also a popular remedy; some people wash them down with a glass of milk. Roasted black sesame seeds ground to a powder and taken with sugar in hot water for breakfast is also known to support good hair and skin health.

The common remedies for hair problems serve to ensure better nutrition to the kidneys, the blood, and the scalp.

Spinach and Black Sesame Seed

One of the best food items for maintaining healthy hair, as recognized all over China, is black sesame seed. Many people eat black sesame seed in large quantities in order to maintain their black, shiny hair. People add the seeds to soups, vegetable dishes, and meats. They make candies with it, or simply chew on black sesame seeds whenever the occasion arises.

This recipe serves to combat hair loss.

¼ cup (50 grams) fresh packed spinach
4 teaspoons (20 grams) black sesame seeds
2 tablespoons (30 milliliters) water

Wash and drain the spinach. Place the spinach, sesame seeds, and water in a wok or small saucepan. Steam over a medium flame for 5 minutes, stirring continuously.

Eat twice daily.

Walnuts and Sesame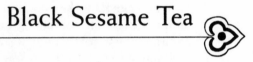

👍👍✌️

1 cup (200 grams) walnut meats, broken into small pieces
1 cup (200 grams) black sesame seeds
1 cup (200 grams) brown sugar

Roast the walnuts and sesame seeds together in a dry frying pan or wok over a low flame for 3 minutes. Stir to ensure that the nuts and seeds do not burn.

Transfer the roasted nuts and seeds to a mortar and pestle. Allow them to cool, then grind to a fine powder. Mix the powder with the sugar, then store in a jar.

Take 1 tablespoon every morning with breakfast.

Black Sesame Tea

👍👍✌️

1 teaspoon (5 grams) black sesame seeds
½ teaspoon (2.5 grams) green tea leaves
1 cup (250 milliliters) water

Roast the sesame seeds for 3 minutes in a dry frying pan over a low flame.

Allow the seeds to cool, then grind them into a powder with a mortar and pestle or a stone grinder. In a cup, mix the powder with the tea leaves.

Bring the water to a boil, then pour into the cup. Brew in hot water for 5 minutes, as you would an ordinary cup of tea.

Spinach Roots, Eggplant, and Black Beans

In some rural areas in the north of China, many people use black beans instead of black sesame seed. The tonifying and ascending Yang qualities, as well as the color of black beans, are said to maintain the hair, making it shiny, black, and healthy. The following recipe comes from Shaanxi province, not far from the Yellow River.

2 cups (500 milliliters) water
2 tablespoons (30 grams) black beans
2 tablespoons (30 grams) spinach root (or the bottom part of the stalk), cut into 1-inch pieces
1 eggplant skin, cut into 1-inch pieces

In a medium saucepan, bring the water to a boil. Add the beans, spinach root, and eggplant skin, and boil over a low flame for 40 minutes, or until the beans are soft enough to eat. Add a little water, if necessary, to ensure that you make a liquid soup rather than a gruel.

Remove from heat. Eat warm. This remedy can be taken as often as you like.

Walnut, Almond, and Jujube Wine

This recipe stimulates blood circulation and improves the complexion. It reinforces qi, and arrests the premature graying of the hair. This recipe also acts as a lung and kidney tonic, thereby curing shortness of breath and lower back pain due to deficiencies in these organs.

¼ cup (50 grams) almond meats
½ cup (100 grams) walnut meats
½ cup (100 grams) jujube (Chinese dates)
8 cups (2 liters) rice wine, or sake

Grind the almonds and the walnuts into a powder using a pestle or a stone grinder. Put the powder and the jujube in a one-gallon bottle. Add the rice wine. Seal the bottle and leave to macerate for at least 20 days before drinking.

Take 2 teaspoons (10 milliliters) two times a day.

The following two remedies help combat hair loss.

Garlic and Honey Poultice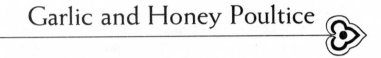

2 heads of garlic, peeled and crushed
2 tablespoons (30 milliliters) honey

In a cup, thoroughly mix the garlic with the honey.

Apply to the affected part of the scalp before going to bed. Wash the poultice off in the morning.

Ginger Head Massage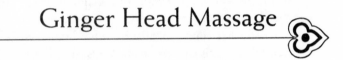

1 large fresh ginger tuber, grated

Squeeze the ginger thoroughly to extract the juice.

Rub the juice into the affected area of the scalp. Leave to dry naturally. Reapply when the scalp has dried. Apply three times at each sitting.

Best results are achieved by massaging the scalp with ginger juice twice a day. It is claimed that, after a week, soft fine hair will begin to grow, and that, within a month, hair growth will be back to normal.

This final remedy is a simple one for strengthening hair and preventing its loss.

Spinach and Carrot Salad

1 cup (200 grams) packed fresh spinach, chopped
1 medium carrot, grated

Mix the spinach and carrot together and eat as salad.

HEADACHE

Headaches can be brought on by so many different factors that it is difficult to prescribe remedies that go to the source of the discomfort. Headaches may be caused by eyestrain, stress, a poor night's sleep, tobacco smoke, toxic fumes, arthritis, a brain tumor, or the common cold. The simplest remedy therefore is to swallow a painkiller and, only if the ache persists, to go to the doctor in order to seek the underlying cause.

In the Chinese countryside, where neither doctors nor painkillers are as easy to come by as in America, other remedies exist. If the cause of the headache is a head cold, one simply cures the cold. Plenty of remedies exist; we refer you to the section on the common cold (pages 98–106) for these.

Headaches without a cold may be alleviated by rubbing eucalyptus oil over the forehead and temples. This gives a cooling sensation that distracts from the pain. Peppermint has a similar effect. You can rub peppermint oil on the temples, dab it under your nose, or drink a cup of peppermint tea.

Another simple headache remedy is to massage the head. Massage is particularly effective if the headache is caused by tension: gently massage the scalp and nape of the neck. A qi gong massage consists of beating on the scalp with the fingers of both hands. Another alternative is to press all your fingers against the scalp and move the entire scalp vigorously backward and forward. Try massaging the temples as well. If no other massage works, press hard with the pads of your thumbs or your two index fingers into the bone of the upper eye socket, close to the top of your nose. Make sure that your fingers are not wet or oily, lest they slip off the bone into the eye itself.

Some of the most effective Chinese food remedies for headaches come in the form of teas.

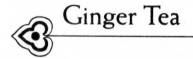

Ginger Tea

Ginger tea is particularly effective for headaches that are due to wind and cold weather.

1½ cups (375 milliliters) water
2 teaspoons (10 grams) fresh ginger, sliced
2 teaspoons (10 grams) brown sugar

In a small saucepan, bring the water to a boil. Add the ginger and sugar and simmer on a low flame for 10 minutes. Transfer the tea to a cup and drink hot.

To be taken three times a day for as long as the headache persists.

Almond and Chrysanthemum Tea

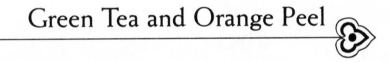

👍👍👍 ✍

Almonds and chrysanthemum flowers have a cooling effect. Combined in a tea, they are effective against headaches due to wind and heat.

1½ cups (375 milliliters) water
1 teaspoon (5 grams) almond meats, ground or chopped
1 teaspoon (5 grams) dry chrysanthemum flowers

In a small saucepan, bring the water to a boil. Add the almonds and chrysanthemum flowers, reduce the flame, and let simmer for 15 minutes.

Remove from heat and drink hot.

Green Tea and Orange Peel

👍👍👍 ✍

This tea is suitable for treating headache associated with nausea and catarrh.

1 teaspoon (5 grams) green tea leaves
1 organic orange peel, chopped
1½ cups (375 milliliters) water

Place the tea leaves, orange peel, and water in a small saucepan. Simmer over a low flame for 10 minutes.

Drink the tea twice a day.

Chrysanthemum Wine

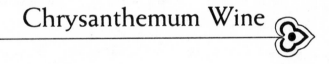

👍👍 ✌

Sometimes wines are prepared for headaches instead of teas.

1 cup (200 grams) dry chrysanthemum flowers
8 cups (2 liters) rice wine, or sake

Place the flowers in a bottle with the wine. Seal the bottle. Let stand to macerate for at least 10 days.

Take 2 or 3 teaspoons twice a day.

Scallion and Cinnamon Congee

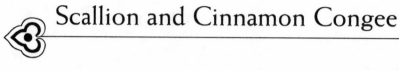

When the body and head ache due to cold and windy climatic conditions, many people in China seek relief in this scallion and cinnamon gruel.

    2 cups (500 milliliters) water
    ¼ cup (50 grams) rice
    10 scallions, cut into ¼-inch segments
    2 teaspoons (10 grams) cinnamon

Place the water, rice, scallions, and cinnamon in a small saucepan. Bring to a boil, cover, then simmer for 20 minutes over a low flame. Add a little water if necessary to form a gruel or congee.

To be taken twice a day with meals.

Mung Bean Congee

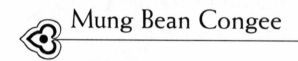

This remedy is recommended for headaches due to summer heat, and overexposure to the sun.

    6 cups (1.5 liters) water
    ¼ cup (50 grams) mung beans
    ½ cup (100 grams) rice

In a medium saucepan, bring water to a boil. Add the mung beans and rice. Boil over a low flame, covered, for 30 minutes, stirring occasionally, to prepare a gruel or congee. Add more hot water if necessary.

Remove from flame. Consume hot or warm.

HEMORRHOIDS

Also known as *piles*, hemorrhoids are caused by a genetic weakness of the veins in the rectum, by sedentary habits, or by constipation. They are characterized by discomfort and sometimes pain, and by frequent bleeding from the rectum during defecation. Hemorrhoids may either be internal or protrude from the body.

The most effective means of preventing piles is to exercise. Although all exercise is beneficial, Chinese qi gong includes a technique whereby the muscles of the rectum are tightened (see the *nei dan* exercises, especially on page 246). This exercise helps to maintain firmness in the rectal muscles with a consequent compression of rectal blood vessels, thus preventing hemorrhoids from developing. A suitable low-fat and low-protein diet of fruits and greens that contain plenty of fiber also works to prevent hemorrhoids.

Wood-ear Mushroom Decoction
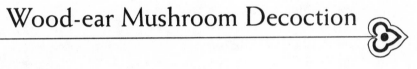

An old remedy for piles is to eat wood-ear mushrooms.

¹/₄ cup (50 grams) wood-ear mushrooms
Water for soaking
2 tablespoons (30 grams) sugar
2 cups (500 milliliters) water

Soak the mushrooms in 1 cup (250 milliliters) of hot water for 1 hour. When you're ready to begin cooking, drain the mushrooms and discard the water.

Put the mushrooms, sugar, and 2 cups (500 milliliters) water into a small saucepan. Bring to a boil. Simmer over a medium flame for 10 minutes to make a decoction.

Divide into three portions. Drink the decoction warm, three times a day.

Escargot

Another ancient Chinese remedy for hemorrhoids is to eat snails.

1 cup (200 grams) bread, torn into large pieces
¹/₂ cup (125 milliliters) vinegar
12 escargot (snails)
4 cups (1 liter) water

To clean the snails, put the bread and vinegar in a container. Add the escargot, cover the container, and refrigerate for 24 hours. The snail will come out of its shell to eat the bread, and the vinegar will disinfect the snail.

When you're ready to cook the snail meat, remove the snails from the container and wash them under running water. Discard the bread. Bring the water to a boil in a medium saucepan. Add the snails in their shells and boil for 10 minutes.

The snails can be eaten in a variety of ways. They may be stir-fried with garlic and herbs, or eaten boiled, dipped in soy sauce and vinegar for flavor. When removing from the shell, be sure to discard the top portion of the snail containing the organs of digestion and excretion.

Mung Bean Soup and Bananas

This high-fiber combination helps prevent hemorrhoids.

1¹/₂ cups (375 milliliters) water
2 tablespoons (30 grams) mung beans
2 ripe bananas

Prepare a decoction by bringing the water to a boil, adding the mung beans, and simmering over a low flame 20 minutes.

Eat twice a day, for breakfast and dinner, together with two bananas.

Hemorrhoids can often be painful. The following two remedies are for pain relief.

❖ Chop and crush 1 medium onion. Transfer the onion to a bowl. Mix with 1 tablespoon (15 milliliters) honey to make a paste. Apply the paste to the hemorrhoid whenever you feel pain.

❖ Squeeze the juice from 3 or 4 cloves of garlic. Dilute the juice in five times the amount of water. Wash the affected area with warm to hot water. Immediately after washing, soak a piece of cotton-wool in the diluted garlic juice and apply to the hemorrhoid. Continue the treatment for as long as necessary.

HEPATITIS

Hepatitis is an inflammation of the liver that may be brought on by either bacteria or a virus. The two most common forms are hepatitis A (infectious) and hepatitis B (serum). The first is usually transmitted through food and is due to poor sanitary conditions. The hepatitis A bacteria reside in feces; the bacteria can pass into drinking water through faulty sewage systems, or into shellfish that breed close to sewage outlets. Serum hepatitis, on the other hand, is caused by direct contact through blood or body fluids, the same way as the HIV virus is spread.

The symptoms of hepatitis include lethargy, nausea, and fever. Urine takes on a reddish brown hue, and the feces become light brown. Recovery is usually spontaneous, although it takes time and plenty of rest for the liver to restore itself. Treatment consists of little more than bed rest and a light diet that does not put strain on the liver.

A person healing from hepatitis should eat plenty of light and energetic foods: ripe fruits, soups, and broth. They should stay away from fat, oil, and milk products, although an exception may be made for light cottage cheese or skimmed milk. An egg a day helps the liver. So does plenty of fluid—drink water and fruit and vegetable juices in large quantities.

Animal liver is a light and energetic food that is ideal for nourishing and rebuilding a damaged liver. Furthermore if it is true, as Chinese theory asserts, that eating animal organs restores health to one's own corresponding organ, liver should do it best of all. Steam, broil, or boil liver, but do not fry it. Fried oil is heavy to digest and will harm the liver at it struggles to recuperate.

In China, hepatitis was not recognized as being due to bacterial and viral infections until recently. Traditional and home remedies thus treat this disease as a genetic weakness of the liver. The following five remedies are aimed specifically at helping the liver to rebuild after the damage caused by the hepatitis. Sugar or honey are used because they provide energy for liver reconstruction.

Soybean Garlic Soup

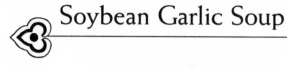

¹/₄ cup (50 grams) soybeans
Water for soaking
3 cups (750 milliliters) water
4 tablespoons (60 grams) sugar, brown or white
1 head of fresh garlic, peeled and crushed

Soak the soybeans overnight in 2 cups (500 milliliters) water. When you are ready to cook, drain the soybeans and discard the water.

In a medium saucepan bring 3 cups water to (750 milliliters) boil. Add the soybeans, cover the pan, and boil over a medium flame for 40 minutes. You want to end up with a watery soup, so add water occasionally if necessary.

Remove from heat and stir in the sugar and crushed garlic.

Divide the soup into two portions. Take hot twice a day. This soup should be taken in combination with one or more of the other therapies described below.

Jujube and Peanuts Sweet

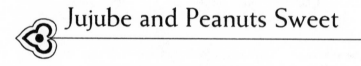

3 cups (750 milliliters) water
¹/₄ cup (50 grams) raw peanuts
10 jujube (Chinese dates)
4 tablespoons (60 grams) brown sugar

In a medium saucepan, bring the water to a boil. Add the peanuts, cover, and simmer over a medium flame for 20 minutes. Add the jujube and sugar. Cover the pan again and simmer for another 15 minutes, until the jujube are cooked. If necessary, occasionally add small quantities of water. The end product should resemble a soup rather than a gruel.

Take 2 tablespoons warm every evening for thirty days, before going to bed.

Celery and Honey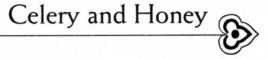

👍👍👍 ✌️

This recipe is a liver reconstructant for infectious hepatitis.

5 stalks of fresh celery, chopped into small pieces
1–2 tablespoons (15–30 milliliters) honey, according to taste
Water for steaming

Using a thin cotton towel, squeeze the celery to extract the juice. Transfer to a bowl for steaming. Add honey.

Put the bowl in a steaming dish (see page 66). Using a pan deep enough to fit your steamer, bring water to a boil. Put the steamer in the pan, cover, and steam for 10 minutes.

Take once a day, preferably in the morning. (You may, as an alternative, heat the celery juice and honey directly in a saucepan for 5 minutes.)

Water Chestnut and Willow Leaf Tea

👍👍👍 ✌️

Water chestnut is a cold and sweet ingredient commonly used in China for indigestion and for liver problems.

5 weeping willow leaves (approximately 6 grams) (collect these
leaves from a nearby tree)
6 water chestnuts, halved
2 cups (500 milliliters) water

Wash the willow leaves. Place the willow leaves and the water chestnuts in a small saucepan with the water. Bring to a boil, then cover and simmer over a low flame for 10 minutes.

Drink frequently as a tea.

Boiled Eggs Flavored with Orange Peel and Anise Seed

3 cups (750 milliliters) water
4 eggs, raw
2 teaspoons (10 grams) organic orange peel, cut
    in $1/2$-inch slices
2 teaspoons (10 grams) ground anise seed

In a medium saucepan, bring the water to a boil. Place the eggs, whole, into the water, along with the orange peel and aniseed. Boil over a medium flame, uncovered, for 10 minutes.

Remove the eggs. Crack the shell, but do not remove the shell. Put the eggs back in the water and simmer over low heat for another 20 minutes.

Remove the eggs from the water and let them cool. Peel the eggs. Eat 2 eggs two times a day.

Pork Gall and Honey

For those adventurous enough to try something unusual, you might take some pork gall with honey. (Anything is worth trying when you are laid up with hepatitis.) Besides strengthening the liver, this recipe also arrests diarrhea.

1 gallbladder of pork, cubed
8 tablespoons (120 grams) honey
Water for steaming

Using a thin cotton towel, squeeze the gallbladder to obtain the gall. Transfer the gall to a ceramic bowl. Stir in the honey.

Put the bowl in a steaming dish (see page 66). Using a pan big enough to fit the steamer, bring water to a boil. Put the steamer in the pan, cover, and steam for 10 minutes. Remove from heat.

Take warm once a day.

HYPERACIDITY

Hyperacidity is a frequent precursor of gastric problems of a more serious nature. To combat hyperacidity, refrain from eating heavy, greasy, sour, or irritating food—that means cutting down on fried foods, heavy roasts, lemon, vinegar and sour fruits, raw vegetables, and green and red chili pepper.

Garlic Pork

A common food remedy for hyperacidity in China is to eat lean pork with garlic.

5 to 7 ounces (150 to 200 grams) lean pork, cut into
¹/₂-inch cubes
1 head of garlic, peeled and crushed
1 cup (250 milliliters) water for steaming

Place the pork in a bowl. Sprinkle the crushed garlic over the pork. Steam together for 30 minutes. Eat as part of your meals.

HYPERTENSION (HIGH BLOOD PRESSURE)

The blood pressure of a healthy adult should ideally be 120 mm Hg (millimeters of mercury), when the lower chamber of the heart contracts to force the blood through the arteries (diastolic pressure), and 80 mm Hg on the rebound, when the same chamber expands to receive blood (systolic pressure). Blood pressure is considered to be "normal" within the range of 90 and 140 mm Hg diastolic, and 60 and 90 mm Hg systolic. Anything higher or lower than that is considered harmful to general health.

Blood pressure is considered to be high when it reads over 140 mm Hg diastolic and 90 mm Hg systolic. Symptoms of high blood pressure are frequent pounding headaches, tension and insomnia, raised arteries at the temple, flushed features, ringing in the ears, ankle swelling, and heart palpitations.

Hypertension arises as a result of the narrowing of the arteries. This may be hereditary, but it may also be due to stress; high cholesterol levels; obesity; the intake of too much alcohol, fat, sugar, or salt; kidney disease; a disease of the endocrine or nervous systems; or to any blockage of the arteries. In the long run, high blood pressure can lead to cardiovascular disease, heart attacks, and stroke. In most cases the cure for hypertension is effected by treating its underlying cause. When this cause is not apparent, as in "essential" or hereditary high blood pressure, it may be treated by the administration of specific drugs or by a combination of diet and exercise.

The first and indispensable dietary measure must be to reduce the intake of sodium, fats, cholesterol, meat, and sugar. A useful second step is to increase the intake of soluble fiber which, it is believed, cleanses the veins and arteries of dangerous cholesterol. Alcohol in doses of one glass of wine or one small shot of Chinese rice wine (or sake) may also combat cholesterol and fat deposits. Any larger amounts, however, harden the arteries and consequently increase blood pressure.

Specific foods used in China to lower blood pressure are kelp and other seaweeds, clams, bean sprouts, bean curd (tofu), celery, garlic, onions, tomatoes, radish, daikon, sesame seeds, sunflower seeds, peanuts, bananas, oranges, persimmon, watermelon (including the rind), potatoes, whole-grain cereals, green tea, and peppermint.

Western studies confirm the validity of all the above products for combating hypertension. Most of them are rich in fiber. Bananas, sunflower seeds, beans, celery, melons and watermelons, oranges, tomatoes, and potatoes—together, with avocados, fish (especially sardines), squash, apricots, and peaches—all contain potassium. Potassium has been shown in numerous studies to neutralize the artery-hardening effects of sodium, as has calcium. Calcium-rich food sources are chickpeas, tofu, beans, greenleaf vegetables, alfalfa sprouts, sunflower seeds, and dairy products. Garlic and onion contain a hormonelike substance called prostaglandin A_1 which lowers blood pressure. It has also been found that vegetarians tend to suffer less frequently from hypertension than do meat eaters.

As well as a high vegetable-fiber intake and a low-fat diet, Chinese treatment of hypertension includes early morning qi gong exercise and brisk walks.

Some specific Chinese food remedies for hypertension are:

- Eat up to 5 ripe bananas a day.
- Eat 1 raw tomato every morning before breakfast. In China, a teaspoon of white sugar is often sprinkled on top.
- Grate 2 cups (400 grams) of fresh radish or daikon. Squeeze out the juice. Drink 1 glass twice a day.
- Eat 2 or 3 raw celery stalks every day, or drink 1 cup (250 milliliters) of raw celery juice.
- Take a glass of celery juice as an afternoon drink, with a handful of sunflower seeds. Take every day for at least one month.

Celery, a diuretic, calms the nerves, warms the stomach, strengthens the liver, and lowers blood pressure. The juice is also considered to be an effective remedy when cooked.

Celery and Rice

👍👍 ✍

¼ cup (50 grams) celery
3 cups (750 milliliters) water
¼ cup (50 grams) rice

Wash the celery, removing the leaves (do not discard them). Chop the celery stalks into ½-inch segments.

Put two saucepans of water on to boil, one containing 2 cups (500 milliliters) of water, the other with 1 cup (250 milliliters). Place the celery and rice in the larger saucepan, cover, and boil for 20 minutes, stirring occasionally, until the rice is soft and mushy. In the meantime, place the celery leaves in the smaller saucepan and boil for 5 minutes.

Add the leaf broth to the congee when the congee is ready.

Take once a day as part of a meal.

Celery and Vegetable Soup

👍👍 ✍

4 cups (1 liter) water
½ cup (100 grams) celery, chopped
5 garlic cloves, peeled and lightly crushed
5 slices onion
5 peeled water chestnuts
1 tomato
1 teaspoon (5 grams) seaweed, optional

In a medium saucepan, bring the water to a boil. Add all ingredients and boil, uncovered, for 15 minutes. Do not add any salt, soy sauce, or stock.

Consume warm before bedtime. Take this remedy for as long as the problem persists.

Note: If you have difficulty finding water chestnuts, you can either dispense with them altogether or use ¼ cup (50 grams) of soybeans or bean sprouts instead.

Boiled Celery Juice

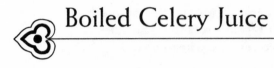

4 cups (1 liter) water
1 cup (200 grams) celery, cut into 1-inch segments

Bring the water to a boil in a medium saucepan. Put the celery into the saucepan and boil for 3 minutes. When it is done, drain the celery and discard the water. Put the celery in a thin cotton towel. Squeeze the celery over a bowl to extract the juice.

Drink the juice either alone or with honey twice a day, morning and evening.

Sugar and Vinegar

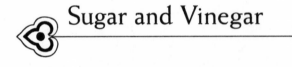

½ cup (125 milliliters) rice vinegar
2 tablespoons (30 grams) rock sugar

Place the vinegar in a small saucepan. Heat over a low flame. When the vinegar is warm, add the sugar. Stir until the sugar melts. Allow to cool.

Sip warm following meals.

Mung Beans and Black Sesame

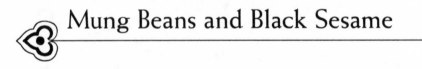

1 cup (200 grams) mung beans
1 cup (200 grams) black sesame seeds

Roast the mung beans and the sesame seeds in a frying pan or wok until they are thoroughly dry. Remove and allow them to cool.

Using a grinding stone or mortar and pestle, grind the roasted beans and seeds into a powder. Take 3 tablespoons (45 grams) of the powder twice a day on cereal or with rice, congee, warm milk, or water.

In China people sometimes collect rather more abstruse ingredients in order to keep their high blood pressure in check. We have included three simple prescriptions using ingredients that might seem unusual but are, in fact, fairly easy to come by.

Watermelon Rind, Corn Threads, and Banana Decoction

2 cups (500 milliliters) water
¼ cup (50 grams) watermelon rind, diced
1 banana, chopped
Threads from the head of 1 ripe corn plant
2 teaspoons (10 grams) brown sugar

In a medium saucepan, bring the water to a boil. Add all the ingredients except the sugar. Simmer over low heat until only 1 cup (250 milliliters) of water is left, approximately 40 minutes.

Remove from heat and add the sugar. Consume warm.

Magnolia Flower Tea

1 cup (250 milliliters) water
1 magnolia *(Magnolia grandiflora)* flower

In a small saucepan, bring the water to a boil. Place the magnolia in a cup and pour the hot water over it. Cover and leave to brew for half an hour.

Drink as a tea.

Earthworm

Although we left this appealing remedy until last, it is in fact one of the most common remedies for hypertension in China. Its efficacy is well proven.

1 earthworm

Wash and dry an earthworm. Chop it into ½-inch segments.

Roast the earthworm for 3 minutes in a dry frying pan. Cool slightly, then grind the segments into a powder.

Take 1 teaspoon of the powder three times a day in hot water, or any other way you may fancy.

HYPOTENSION (LOW BLOOD PRESSURE)

Low blood pressure (lower than 90 mm Hg diastolic and 60 mm Hg systolic—see page 145) leads to sleepiness, weakness, headaches, dizziness, insomnia, tiring easily, lack of concentration, chest pains, and feelings of suffocation. People with very low blood pressure faint easily when standing up suddenly; they are usually pale, sweat profusely, and have a slow heartbeat.

According to Chinese medicine, low blood pressure is due to weak Yang and qi. It is usually accompanied by a weak spleen and stomach. It tends to occur in sedentary intellectual workers, and in elderly people with heart ailments.

Remedies are to eat well and to exercise. The following specific cures might also help.

❖ Eat beef any way you like it. In China it is usually eaten in a stew.
❖ Chew a piece of raw, fresh ginger as you would a candy. You can also add slices of ginger to your soups, teas, or stews. Take three or four a day.
❖ Two tablespoons of sugar in a glass of wine taken twice a day guarantees an increase in blood pressure. Any wine will do.

Tangerine Peel, Walnut, and Licorice Decoction

👍👍✌️

2 cups (500 milliliters) water
1 tablespoon (15 grams) organic tangerine peel, chopped
4 or 5 walnut meats
1 teaspoon (5 grams) pure licorice, or 1 inch of a licorice twig

In a small saucepan, bring the water to a boil. Add all the ingredients and stew over a low flame for 15 minutes.

Drink warm twice a day, morning and evening.

INDIGESTION

Indigestion is due either to a weak stomach and spleen—in Chinese terms, a deficient Earth function—or to grave mistakes in eating habits. You might be eating too fast, talking while you eat, or eating too much or out of season. Please refer to chapter 3 for more information on what you might be doing wrong. Once you have become aware of any errors in your eating habits, the first step is to correct them. If, in spite of your attentiveness, you continue to suffer from indigestion, you might wish to try dissolving 1 teaspoon (5 grams) of ground cinnamon in a glass of warm water. You may drink this three times a day, with meals, as an aid to digestion. Or try one or more of the following traditional remedies.

Tangerine Peel and Ginger Tea

2 teaspoons (10 grams) finely minced organic tangerine peel
2 teaspoons (10 grams) finely minced fresh ginger
1 teaspoon (5 grams) sugar, brown or white
1 cup (250 milliliters) water

In a small saucepan bring the water to a boil. Place the tangerine peel and the ginger in a cup with the sugar, and pour the boiling water over them. Brew for 10 minutes.

Drink warm as a tea. This tea may be taken up to three times a day.

Ginger and Nutmeg Decoction

This remedy strengthens the spleen and stomach; it is commonly used in China to eliminate intestinal worms.

1 cup (250 milliliters) water
1 teaspoon (5 grams) sliced fresh ginger
1½ teaspoons (8 grams) ground nutmeg

In a small saucepan, bring the water to a boil. Add the ginger and nutmeg. Cover and simmer over a low flame for 15 minutes.

Drink ½ cup (125 milliliters) of the decoction twice a day before meals.

Water Chestnut and Radish Juice

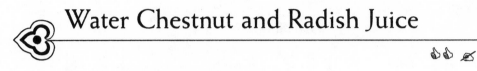

20 water chestnuts, sliced
1 cup (200 grams) radish, sliced

Using a thin cotton towel, squeeze the water chestnuts and the radish to extract their juices. Mix the juices in a small saucepan. Warm the juice, but do not allow it to boil.

Drink warm as a tea, following meals.

Peppered Jujube

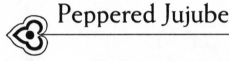

1 teaspoon (5 grams) black peppercorns
10 jujube (Chinese dates) sliced in half
1½ cups (375 milliliters) water
5 slices dried ginger

Using a grinding stone or mortar and pestle, grind the pepper into a medium-grain powder.

In a small saucepan, bring the water to a boil. Add the pepper and jujube. Cover and simmer for 15 minutes.

Drink warm or cool. To be taken after meals once or twice a day.

INSOMNIA

Insomnia may result from a genetic predisposition, a stressful lifestyle, or worry. It may depend on dietary deficiencies such as a lack of calcium or magnesium, or it may be caused by the consumption of too much caffeine. Whatever the causes, there are several measures you can take to counteract chronic insomnia.

The first thing you should do is stop taking coffee, tea, colas, and other stimulants in the afternoons and evenings. You can drink a glass of milk before going to bed—don't put chocolate or cocoa in it, though, as they too are mild stimulants.[9] You can, like the majority of Chinese people, wash your feet in hot water and then massage the soles of your feet every night just before going to bed. You can make love before going to sleep—both male and female orgasms stimulate the secretion of a morphinelike substance in the brain.

You can also practice relaxing. Regular exercise and qi gong deep breathing will help you to relax. Try standing in the qi gong position for fifteen to twenty minutes two to three hours before going to bed (see page 245). Once in bed, ten to fifteen minutes of slow, deep breathing while lying on your back should ensure a good night's rest.

If, however, you still cannot sleep, try the following Chinese remedy:

1. Stand in the qi gong breathing position with knees bent and arms outstretched until you begin to sweat. Ten to twenty minutes should suffice.
2. Walk between one and two hundred paces, swinging your arms vigorously with each pace.
3. Wash your feet and hands in hot water.
4. Massage the underside of your feet by pressing one hundred times on the soft point in the center of the foot, where the toe bones meet and the arch begins.
5. Go back to bed and try sleeping again.

The following are a few other traditional Chinese remedies for insomnia.

❖ Chop an onion and keep it in a jar. When you cannot sleep, open the jar and inhale through your nose. The onion fumes send you to sleep within fifteen minutes.
❖ Eat 20 to 30 sunflower seeds before bed.
❖ Brew 1 tablespoon (15 grams) of wheat bran in hot water, as if you were making a tea. Filter and drink before bed.

Scallion and Jujube Decoction

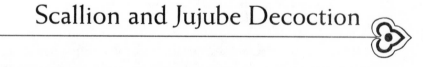

This bedtime decoction frequently accompanies, and is said to enhance the effects of, the foot-soaking ritual described above.

> **4 cups (1 liter) water**
> **8 white heads of scallions, thinly sliced**
> **15 jujube (Chinese dates)**
> **1 teaspoon (5 grams) brown sugar**

In a medium saucepan, bring the water to a boil. Add the scallion, jujube, and sugar. Cover and simmer over a medium flame for 30 minutes. Drink 1 cup of the decoction warm, before going to bed.

Millet Broth and Egg Patty

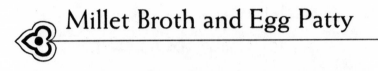

1½ cups (375 milliliters) water
4 tablespoons (60 grams) millet
1 egg

In a small saucepan, bring the water to a boil. Add the millet and turn the heat to low. Simmer for 30 minutes, uncovered, until the soup becomes a gruel. Stir so as not to allow the millet to clump or burn. Add a little water occasionally if the liquid is evaporating too quickly. When you have a creamy broth, remove from heat. Strain the liquid part into a bowl.

Beat the egg in a separate bowl. Pour the liquid from the millet broth and the beaten egg into a small frying pan or wok. Heat the mixture for 5 minutes over a medium flame, stirring until it solidifies. Remove pan from heat.

Eat warm as part of dinner.

Walnuts and Sesame Seeds

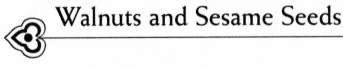

¼ cup (50 grams) walnut meats
¼ cup (50 grams) black sesame seeds
1 tablespoon (15 grams) sugar, brown or white

Roast the walnuts and sesame seeds in a dry frying pan or wok over a low flame. Allow the nuts and seeds to cool, then transfer to a pestle or stone grinder and grind to a medium-fine powder.

Mix the powder with sugar. Take 1 tablespoon (15 grams) two hours before bedtime.

Steamed Rolls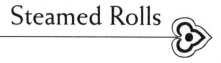

Some recipes may be taken during the day, well before bedtime. These steamed rolls, for instance, are usually eaten for breakfast.

¹/₂ cup (100 grams) wheat flour
2 tablespoons (30 milliliters) water
3 tablespoons (45 milliliters) sesame oil
Water for steaming

Mix the flour with the water and the sesame oil. Roll the dough into two round buns.

Transfer the buns to a ceramic bowl or steaming dish (see page 66). Using a pan deep enough to fit your steamer, bring water to a boil. Put the steamer in the pan, cover, and steam for 20 minutes.

Remove from heat. Take this remedy once a day for a week.

Goats' Hearts and Roses

This recipe may be difficult to execute unless you live on a farm or happen to know a butcher who can provide the goat's heart. If goat heart proves too difficult to come by, you might wish to try the recipe with lamb instead.

This remedy counteracts insomnia by strengthening the heart and blood circulation. It is also recommended for depression.

1 cup (250 milliliters) water
2 teaspoons (10 grams) salt
Fresh petals from 1 rose (approximately ¹/₄ cup or 50 grams)
2 ounces (60 grams) goat's heart, cubed

In a small saucepan, bring the water and salt to a boil. Add the rose petals. Simmer over a low flame for 10 minutes.

Put the meat in the rose water. Leave to marinate for 15 minutes. Skewer the meat and roast it over an open fire, or barbecue for 15 to 20 minutes. While cooking, brush frequently with the rose water.

Eat as part of dinner.

MENOPAUSE

Menopause is the cessation of menstruation. Although it is not accompanied by any physical deterioration, the hormonal changes involved do take their toll on the well-being of many women.

The characteristic symptoms of menopause are brought about by the decline in the body's production of the hormone estrogen. The decrease in estrogen disturbs the function of the hypothalamus, which is responsible for regulating body heat and metabolism—hence the characteristic "hot flashes" and the increase in weight frequently accompanying menopause. The hormonal imbalance also takes its toll emotionally, many women feeling that age has finally caught up with them. Until recently, menopause was regarded as the definitive end of sexual activity—of youth, childbearing, and vigor: the conclusion of the "prime" of life and the beginning of old age. It is small wonder, therefore, that many women go through a period of deep depression with the onset of menopause.

In China, youth is not as prized as in the West. Indeed, our culture looks up to older people, paying heed to what they tell us. One of our most common terms of respect is the prefix *lao*, which means "old." We use this whenever we speak or refer to someone who we respect and who is older than ourselves.

As a consequence of this respect, the postmenopause years are regarded with equanimity. It is a time of freedom from the burdens and responsibilities of childbearing and child rearing. Women are at last able to enjoy the fruits of their labors and to achieve a measure of respect both from within the family and from society. It is little wonder, therefore, that in China a woman's years of maturity can be the happiest of her life.

Be this as it may, it is undeniable that the physical symptoms of menopause can, at the very least, be unpleasant. In China several remedies exist that aim toward reducing the effects of hormonal imbalance, such as sleeplessness and irritability. The first one is a classic remedy that may also be used as a generic tonic for the nervous system. You may have to visit an herbalist or a Chinese food store to obtain the licorice and jujube, or you may purchase it by mail order. Twig licorice is to be preferred. However, if this is difficult to come by, ordinary black unsweetened licorice may be used. If that, too, is unavailable, you can resort to the candy variety.

Licorice, Jujube, and Wheat

¹/₄ cup (50 grams) wheat berries
Water for soaking
3 cups (750 milliliters) water
1 tablespoon (15 grams) licorice
10 jujube (Chinese dates)

Soak the wheat berries overnight in 2 cups (500 milliliters) of water. When you're ready to cook, drain the berries and discard the water.

In a medium saucepan, bring 3 cups (750 milliliters) of water to a boil. Add the licorice. Cover the pan and simmer on a low flame for 20 minutes.

Discard the solid licorice and keep only the liquid decoction. Now add the wheat and the jujube. Cover the pan and cook over a medium flame in the licorice juice for 40 minutes, until the wheat is edible.

Eat as you would a porridge.

Two more recipes based on the tonifying effects of jujube follow.

Adzuki Beans and Jujube Congee

4 cups (1 liter) water
¹/₂ cup (100 grams) adzuki beans
10 jujube (Chinese dates)
¹/₄ cup (50 grams) rice

In a medium saucepan, bring the water to a boil. Add the beans, jujube, and rice. Cover and simmer over a low to medium flame for 30 minutes. Stir, adding water if necessary until ingredients are cooked.

Consume warm as a porridge. This remedy can be taken as often as you like, as part of a meal.

157

Jujube and Pork Rind

10 jujube (Chinese dates), split in half
2 ounces (60 grams) pork rind, finely chopped
Water for steaming

Place the pork and jujube in a ceramic bowl or steaming dish (see page 66). Using a pan deep enough to fit your steamer, bring water to a boil. Place the steamer in the pan and cover. Steam for 30 minutes.

Remove from heat. Divide the dish into three portions. Consume them all in one day, at four-hour intervals.

Boiled Jellyfish

Cold jellyfish is a classic hors d'oeuvre in China. We generally eat it cured in vinegar. Cured jellyfish can be purchased in most Chinese food stores in America.

5 ounces (155 grams) jellyfish
3 cups (750 milliliters) water
Salt to taste
Soy sauce, as garnish
Vinegar, as garnish

Wash the jellyfish thoroughly.

Bring the water to a boil in an earthenware pot (or medium saucepan—the earthenware pot is not indispensable). Put the jellyfish in the pot and boil over a medium flame, uncovered, for 20 minutes, until over two-thirds of the water has evaporated and you are left with a little under 1 cup of liquid.

Remove from heat. Add salt to the broth to taste. Slice the jellyfish, and garnish with soy sauce and vinegar.

Drink the broth hot once a day for five days. After that, take it once every ten days until the unpleasant symptoms of menopause have disappeared. Eat the jellyfish as part of a meal.

Seaweed Soup

👍👍👍 ✌

Seaweed is another Chinese remedy for alleviating the unpleasant symptoms connected with menopause. Unless taken from a polluted sea, seaweed is one of the healthiest sources of minerals available. It nourishes the blood and works wonders for pains in the joints and the back.

You can either buy dried seaweed or pick your own on an unpolluted beach. In the latter case, make sure the seaweed is fresh before consuming it. Roast the fresh seaweed over a charcoal fire; this serves to dry the seaweed. Do not cook or burn it. Once dried, you can add the seaweed to a stew or, indeed, to any dish of your choosing. In China, we usually eat seaweed in soup.

1 cup (250 milliliters) water
2 tablespoons (30 grams) dried seaweed
1 teaspoon (5 milliliters) soy sauce
$^1/_2$ teaspoon (2.5 grams) pepper

In a small saucepan, bring the water to a boil. Place the seaweed, soy sauce, and pepper in a bowl. Pour the hot water into the bowl.

Consume hot or warm, as often as you like.

MENSTRUAL CRAMPS (DYSMENORRHEA)

Painful cramps felt just before or during menstruation are usually caused by an excessive release of the hormonelike substance prostaglandin, which causes the uterus to contract vigorously before a period. Therapy usually consists of the administration of drugs that block the formation of prostaglandin.

If you dislike the idea of interfering with the functions of the body by taking drugs, four Chinese natural remedies may be useful in combating the pain. One is an external application to the abdomen; the other three are decoctions or teas.

Ginger, Onion, and Salt Compress

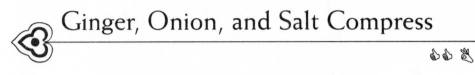

> 1 cup (225 grams) fresh ginger, finely chopped
> ½ onion, crushed
> 1 pound (500 grams) salt

Mix the ginger and onion with the salt. Roast the mixture in a dry frying pan or wok for 10 minutes.

Pack the heated ingredients inside a thin towel. While hot, apply to the abdominal area. It is best to lie on one's back during the application.

Apply twice a day for three days before the onset of menstruation.

Ginger and Sugar Decoction

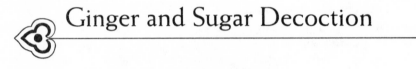

> 1½ cups (375 milliliters) water
> 5 slices (15 grams) fresh ginger
> 1 tablespoon (15 grams) brown sugar

In a small saucepan, bring the water to a boil. Add the ginger and sugar, lower the flame, and simmer, covered, for 15 minutes.

Drink the decoction warm to hot twice a day, just before the onset of the period until the end of menstruation.

Ginger, Scallion, and Pepper Tea

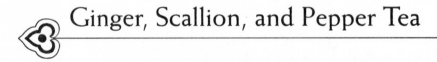

> 1 cup (250 milliliters) water
> 1 2-ounce piece (60 grams) ginger, sliced thin
> 5 white heads of scallion, chopped
> ½ cup (100 grams) brown sugar
> 1 teaspoon (5 grams) black pepper

In a small saucepan, bring the water to a boil. Mix the ginger and scallion with the sugar. Add to the water, cover, and simmer over a low flame for 10 minutes.

Remove from heat, pour into a cup, add the pepper, and drink hot.

To be taken three times a day prior to and during your menstrual period.

Rose Tea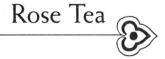

👍👍👍 ✌️

1 cup (250 milliliters) water
Fresh petals from 1 rose (approximately ¹/₄ cup or 50 grams)

In a small saucepan, bring the water to a boil.

Place the petals in a cup and pour the boiling water over them. Steep for 5 to 10 minutes before drinking.

To be taken five days before the onset of your period, until bleeding stops. This therapy is recommended for three successive months.

NAUSEA AND VOMITING

In the West, a common remedy for nausea and vomiting is to drink warm lemon juice with sugar. Since lemons are not common in China, most Chinese remedies include the use of fresh ginger.

Ginger and Honey Tea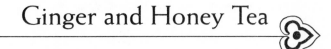

👍👍👍 ✌️

1 6-ounce (180-gram) piece of ginger, grated
2 tablespoons (30 milliliters) honey
Water for steaming
2 cups (500 milliliters) water

Using a thin cotton towel, squeeze the ginger to extract 4 tablespoons (60 milliliters) of juice. Transfer the juice and honey to a ceramic bowl, and put the bowl in a steaming dish (see page 66).

Using a pan deep enough to fit your steamer, bring water to a boil. Place the steamer in the pan and steam for 5 minutes, until warm.

Heat 2 cups (500 milliliters) of water in a separate pan. Pour the ginger juice and honey and the warm water into a cup. Sip slowly.

Ginger and Sugarcane Juice

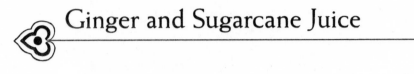

This recipe is recommended for both chronic nausea due to stomach problems and nausea due to pregnancy.

3 tablespoons (45 grams) grated fresh ginger
1 cup (250 milliliters) sugarcane juice

Using a thin cotton towel, squeeze the ginger to extract the juice. Add the ginger juice to the sugarcane juice. Stir well.
Sip slowly.

Ginger and Tangerine Decoction

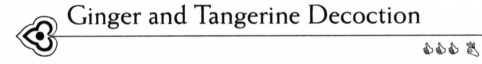

1 organic tangerine peel, cut into ¹/₂-inch slices
1 teaspoon (5 grams) sliced fresh ginger
1¹/₂ cups (375 milliliters) water

Place the tangerine and ginger in a pot with the water. Bring to a boil, then simmer, covered, over a low flame for 15 minutes.
Drink 1 cup, hot, twice a day.

Ginger and Vinegar

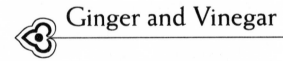

3 slices fresh ginger
¹/₄ cup (60 milliliters) vinegar
1 cup (250 milliliters) water
1 teaspoon (5 grams) brown sugar

Soak the ginger in the vinegar for at least 6 hours. Drain.
In a small saucepan, bring the water to a boil. Place the ginger in a cup. Add the boiling water and sugar.
Allow to steep for 5 minutes before drinking slowly.

Ginger, Potato, and Orange Juice

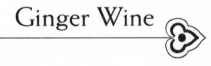

👍👍👍 ✌️

This ginger juice preparation should be taken with every meal in order to inhibit the sense of nausea.

2 teaspoons (10 grams) grated fresh ginger
1 potato, peeled and grated
1 orange, peeled and sectioned

Using a thin cotton towel, squeeze the ginger, the potato, and the orange to extract their juices.

Store in a small bottle and refrigerate. Take 1 tablespoon (15 grams) before every meal.

Ginger Wine

👍👍 ✌️

¹⁄₂ cup (125 grams) fresh ginger, finely minced
¹⁄₄ cup (60 grams) organic orange peel, finely minced
1 cup (250 grams) sugar, brown or white
4 cups (1 liter) rice wine, or sake

Place the ginger, orange peel, and sugar in a bottle with the rice wine. Seal the bottle and leave to macerate for at least 10 days.

Take 2 teaspoons once a day after lunch or dinner.

Some remedies for nausea that utilize ingredients other than fresh ginger follow.

❖ Mix 2–3 tablespoons (30–45 grams) of fresh daikon juice with 2 teaspoons (10 grams) of brown sugar. Add to a cup of hot water and drink slowly.
❖ Decoct 2 teaspoons (10 grams) of caraway seed with 1 teaspoon (5 grams) of dried ginger and 1 teaspoon (5 grams) of cinnamon in 1¹⁄₂ cups (375 milliliters) of water. Simmer for 15 to 20 minutes. Drink warm to control hiccuping and vomiting.
❖ A good remedy for nausea due to changing weather, excessive tiredness, and cold is to boil 4 ounces (125 grams) of tofu in water for 20 minutes. Add a little salt and eat warm.

❖ Boil 12–20 cloves in a small saucepan with 1 cup (250 milliliters) water for 5 minutes. Remove from heat and add ¹/₂ teaspoon (2.5 grams) of black tea leaves. Brew for 5 to 10 minutes and drink as an ordinary tea. Clove tea relieves nausea, excessive gastric secretion, and hiccuping.
❖ In the south of China, where pineapples are common, a few slices of pineapple or sips of pineapple juice are everyday remedies for nausea and vomiting.

OBESITY

Any definition of obesity is probably more cultural and personal than objective. During the Tang dynasty in China, a round, full face and body were the epitome of beauty. The large-paunched laughing Buddha placed at the entrance of Buddhist temples in China represents health and abundance; that is why he is there. Even today, when international standards of health and beauty dictate a slim waistline, people in China still consider a few extra pounds to be a sign of health and prosperity.

Having said that, there is no doubt that too much extra weight is harmful. Extra pounds put stress on the skeleton as well as on the heart and circulation. They lead to exhaustion, circulation problems, lower resistance to diseases, kidney problems, diabetes, and, all too often, an early death.

Chinese doctors believe that the tendency to put on weight comes primarily from genetics—some people burn up calories more slowly than others. However, no matter what one's genetic propensities may be, putting on weight is, in 95 percent of all instances, due to personal habits.* In other words, it is caused by nei yin, or endogenous factors: poor eating and exercise habits, a stressful lifestyle, and the seven pathogenic emotions.

People overeat and do not exercise for a variety of reasons. They may be lazy; they may have low blood pressure, which can engender lethargy. They may be depressed or suffering from stress or anxiety. Which leads our discussion to the other cause of obesity—an excess of the seven pathogenic emotions, which include anger, melancholy, worry, grief, fear, fright, and joy.

The first step in dealing with obesity is, therefore, to put some order in one's life. Diminish stress and distress; eliminate those situations that lead to anger, worry, and fear. Try not to indulge in melancholy. Be cheerful, but don't enjoy yourself too much either, remembering that too much joy is also known to take its toll on the body. Above all, try not to overeat.

Qi gong exercise is known to help against obesity. Besides burning off a few calories, qi gong deep breathing appears to readjust the hunger-regulating mechanisms of the hypothalamus, enabling you to stop craving food simply because your hypothalamus does not know that you have eaten enough. Furthermore,

---

* About 5 percent of all cases of obesity are due to hormonal imbalances or glandular defects.

regular qi gong exercise breeds discipline, and discipline allows you to keep up the resolve necessary to cut down on calories. Finally, exercise has a calming effect on the emotions, thus balancing the endogenous factors responsible for obesity.

Certain foods are said to burn fat and calories. Others detoxify the body of excess fat. The following remedies are some of the best:

- Eat 1 whole raw cucumber twice a day. Cucumber cools the body and rids toxins from the blood.
- Eat 1 raw daikon every day. Daikon exerts the same cooling and detoxifying effects as cucumber.
- Wash and shred 4 ounces (125 grams) of fresh lotus leaves. Place the shredded leaves in a pot with 1¹/₂ cups of water and boil over a low flame for 15 to 20 minutes. Drink the decoction once a day. (Lotus leaves can be found in many Chinese food stores.)
- Boil ¹/₂ ounce (15 grams) of corn silk in a pot with 1¹/₂ cups (375 milliliters) of water over a low flame for 15 minutes. Consume as a tea. Corn silk burns fats.
- Frequent tea drinking burns excessive fat in the bloodstream and tissues. Green tea without any additive is to be preferred to red or black teas.

Daikon and Mushroom Decoction

¹/₂ cup (100 grams) wood-ear mushrooms
Water for soaking
1 cup (200 grams) daikon, sliced
3 cups (750 milliliters) water
Salt to taste

Soak the wood-ear mushrooms in 2 cups (500 milliliters) hot water for 1 hour, or until they are soft.

Place the mushrooms and daikon in a pot with 3 cups (750 milliliters) water. Boil over a low flame for 15 to 20 minutes.

Remove from heat. Add salt to taste.

Drink hot twice a day, for as long as you like.

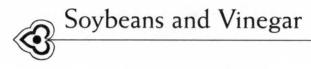

Soybeans and Vinegar

2 cups (400 grams) soybeans
2 cups (500 milliliters) vinegar

Roast the soybeans in a dry frying pan or wok over a medium flame for 5 minutes, or until the beans are a golden brown. Let the soybeans cool, then pour back into a 1-liter bottle.

Fill the bottle with vinegar. Leave in the refrigerator for 5 days. Eat 1 teaspoon (5 grams) of beans two times a day, morning and evening.

PREGNANCY

Nausea and Vomiting

Most women experience at least some nausea during the first months of pregnancy. In fact, the huge number of recipes that exist in China for this condition attests to how common morning sickness is. We have selected those remedies that are easiest to prepare.

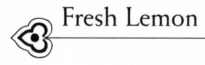

Fresh Lemon

3–4 medium lemons, peeled and seeded
1 cup (200 grams) sugar

Cut the lemons into 1-inch segments. Place in a small saucepan. Stir in the sugar. Let stand for 12 hours.

Heat the lemon-sugar mixture over a low flame for 10 minutes, in order to dry the juice. Take 1–2 teaspoons (5–10 grams) of the dry lemon every time you feel nauseous.

Kiwi and Fresh Ginger Juice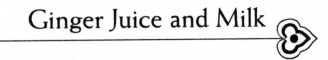

👍👍👍 ✌️

This recipe is relatively new to the folk remedy medicine chest, as kiwi have only recently arrived in China. Ginger is a traditional nausea suppressant, and kiwi has an acidic tang to it that is known to give physical relief from the urge to vomit.

1 kiwi, peeled and chopped
2 teaspoons (10 grams) ginger, grated

Using a thin cotton towel, squeeze the kiwi and the ginger to extract the juice. Mix the juices.
 Take two times a day, morning and evening.

Ginger Juice and Milk

👍👍👍 ✌️

The following remedy inhibits the urge to vomit and is sufficiently nutritious to replenish any solid food that one may throw up or be unable to swallow due to nausea.

1 cup (250 milliliters) milk
2 teaspoons (10 milliliters) fresh ginger juice
4 teaspoons (20 grams) sugar, white or brown

Mix the ingredients and bring them to a boil in a small saucepan. When the milk rises, remove from the heat.
 Drink warm, two times a day.

Other remedies using ginger as a nausea suppressant follow.

- Decoct 2 teaspoons (10 grams) fresh ginger and 1 tablespoon (15 grams) brown sugar in 1¹⁄₂ cups (375 milliliters) water, simmering for 15 minutes. Take this decoction two times a day, morning and evening.
- Add 1 tablespoon (15 milliliters) ginger juice to a glass of sugarcane juice. Fresh sugarcane is preferable but if it is unavailable, canned juice will do. Mix well and sip slowly. This is a good remedy for nausea and vomiting, as well as for a poor appetite.
- Mix 1 tablespoon (15 milliliters) ginger juice with 2 tablespoons (30 milliliters) honey and 3 tablespoons (45 milliliters) water. Warm them by steaming in a ceramic bowl and steamer (see page 66). Take three times a day.

❖ Remove the peel from 1 organic orange. Cut the peel into fine slices. Put the orange peel and 2 tablespoons (30 grams) of chopped, fresh ginger in a cup. Pour freshly boiled water into the cup and leave to brew for 5 or 10 minutes. Add sugar to taste, and drink as a tea.

The following are simple remedies that do not depend on ginger for suppressing nausea.

Chive Tea

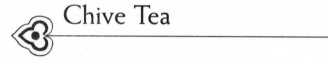

4 or 5 chives, chopped
1½ cups (375 milliliters) water

In a small saucepan, bring the water to a boil. Add the chives and simmer over a low flame for 10 minutes.

Drink the decoction hot in the mornings, or whenever you feel nauseous.

Egg Cooked in Vinegar

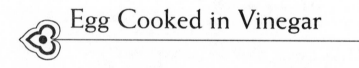

1 raw egg
4 tablespoons (70 milliliters) vinegar
2 tablespoons (30 grams) white sugar

Beat the egg in a bowl.

In a small saucepan, bring the vinegar to a boil. Turn the heat to low and add the sugar. When the sugar has melted, pour in the beaten egg. *Do not stir.* Cook the egg for 4 minutes.

Remove the egg with a slotted spoon.

Eat one egg per day.

Apple Peel and Rice Decoction

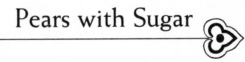

This is a nutritious, nausea-suppressing remedy that is easy to prepare.

> 2 tablespoons (30 grams) rice
> ¼ cup (50 grams) organic apple peel, cut into 2-inch pieces
> 2 cups (500 milliliters) water

Roast the rice in a dry frying pan or wok over a low flame for 3 minutes, until it is golden brown.

Place the apple peel and rice in a medium pot with the water. Simmer over a low flame for 20 minutes.

Drink hot as a tea whenever you feel nauseous.

Coughing During Pregnancy

Some women suffer from frequent coughing during pregnancy. The reason for this is that the growing fetus puts pressure on the lower diaphragm, thus irritating the lungs and giving rise to the urge to cough. According to Chinese doctors, this irritation occurs only in women who are weak in Yin. During pregnancy, qi and blood concentrate around the womb, thus reducing their effectiveness in the upper body. The lungs and bronchial passages are thus undernourished, and so become susceptible to any slight irritation.

In order to correct this problem, one should consume foods that strengthen Yin and qi. A tasty breakfast dish with these Yin- and qi-enhancing effects is pears with sugar.

Pears with Sugar

> 2 pears, cut into small pieces
> 2 cups (500 milliliters) water
> 1 tablespoon (15 grams) brown sugar

Place the pears in a small saucepan with the water and the sugar. Bring to a boil, then simmer for 20 minutes over a low flame.

Drink the decoction and eat the pears. To be taken every morning for breakfast.

Abdominal Pains During Pregnancy

Another frequent problem that arises during pregnancy is pain in the abdomen. According to Chinese theory, abdominal pains during pregnancy are due to the stagnation of qi in the womb and its poor circulation around the rest of the abdomen. The cure is to nourish the qi and the blood. Two simple recipes serve this purpose.

❖ Cut 1 daikon into ¼-inch slices. Eat five slices at a time, sprinkling them with a little sugar according to taste. To be eaten three times a day with meals.
❖ Prepare a congee by mixing ½ cup (100 grams) of sliced, mature pumpkin with 3 cups (750 milliliters) water, 2 tablespoons (30 grams) rice, and 4 teaspoons (20 grams) sugar. Simmer over a low flame for 20 minutes. This congee should be eaten warm two times a day.

Insufficient Breast Milk

The problem of insufficient breast milk after childbirth is a common one in China, if we are to judge by the number of recipes that aim to increase breast milk secretion.

Poor lactation can be caused by stress, ill health, general weakness, or an irregular suckling pattern. According to Chinese theory, poor lactation results from weak qi and blood circulation. Accompanying symptoms are soft breasts (and therefore a lack of swelling and pain in these glands) facial pallor, bouts of dizziness, tinnitus, lack of appetite, sweating at night, and irritability. The remedy is to strengthen the mother by means of nutritious and protein-rich foods. One very simple way of doing this is to eat ½ cup (100 grams) of boiled green peas twice a day, on an empty stomach. Other examples of such nutritious food remedies follow.

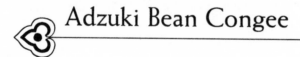

Adzuki Bean Congee

½ cup (100 grams) adzuki beans
½ cup (100 grams) rice
4 cups (1 liter) water

Place the adzuki beans, rice, and water in a medium saucepan. Bring to a boil, then cover and simmer for 20 to 30 minutes over a low flame. Stir occasionally so the rice does not stick to the pan.

To be consumed warm once or twice a day.

Lettuce and Licorice Congee

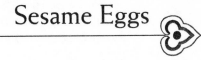

👍👍👍 ✋

4 large leaves of lettuce, chopped
1 teaspoons (5 grams) licorice
4 cups (1 liter) water
½ cup (100 grams) rice

Place the lettuce, licorice, and water in a medium saucepan. Bring to a boil, then simmer over a low flame for 10 to 15 minutes.

Remove from heat and cool slightly. When it is cool enough to work with, pass the mixture through a sieve to remove some of the solid ingredients.

Transfer the liquid back to the saucepan. Add the rice. Simmer over a low flame for 20 minutes, stirring occasionally, to make a rice congee.

Take the congee three times a day for five days.

Sesame Eggs

👍👍👍 ✋

1 cup (200 grams) black sesame seeds
2 teaspoons (10 grams) salt
2 eggs
2 cups (500 milliliters) water

Roast the sesame seeds in a dry frying pan or wok over a low flame for 1 minute, until you can smell the distinct odor of sesame. Add salt, and roast for another 30 seconds.

Place the eggs in a small saucepan with water. Bring to a boil, then continue to boil over medium heat for 15 minutes.

Remove from heat. Allow the eggs to cool, then remove the shells and cut the eggs into segments. Mix the eggs with the sesame, and consume warm.

Tofu with Sugar

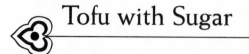

4 ounces (125 grams) tofu, cut into 1-inch cubes
½ cup (100 grams) brown sugar
3 cups (750 milliliters) water

Place the tofu in a medium saucepan together with the sugar and water. Bring to a boil, then simmer for 20 minutes, uncovered, over low heat. Remove from the heat. Consume warm.

Papaya Fish

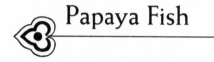

2 tablespoons cooking oil
1 tablespoon (15 grams) sliced fresh ginger
Pinch of salt
1 carp or trout, approximately 1 pound (500 grams), cleaned
5 cups (1.25 liters) water
1 cup (200 grams) papaya, cut into 8 slices

Heat the oil in a wok. Throw in the ginger with a pinch of salt. When the ginger begins to crackle, put the fish in the pan. Fry the fish evenly, 5 minutes on each side, until the skin is crisp.

Bring the water to boil in a large terracotta pot. (If a terracotta pot is unavailable, use an ordinary saucepan.) Place the papaya and the fish in the boiling water, and allow to simmer on a low flame, covered, for 30 minutes.

This dish should be eaten at least once a day, until breast milk flows abundantly. If lactation is particularly scant, eat this dish twice a day, for lunch and for dinner.

Pied du Porc Soup

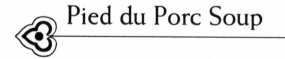

Pied du porc, otherwise called trotters or pig's foot, *is a Chinese peasant dish that was much loved by Chairman Mao.*

1 gallon (4 liters) water
1 pig's foot
5 teaspoons (25 grams) black sesame seeds

In a large soup pot, bring the water to a boil. Put the pig's foot in the pot, turn the heat to low, and simmer, covered, for 1¹/₂ to 2 hours, adding water occasionally as necessary.

In the meantime, roast the sesame seeds over a low flame in a dry wok or frying pan for 3 minutes. Grind the seeds to a medium-fine powder.

When the pig's foot is done, transfer the broth to a bowl. Sprinkle the sesame powder over the soup.

Take a bowl of the soup with meals, three times a day.

Peanuts and Soymilk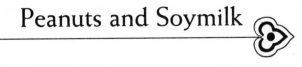

👍👍👍 ✌️

> **12 raw peanuts, shelled**
> **Water for soaking**
> **1 cup (250 milliliters) soymilk**

Soak the peanuts in hot water for 20 minutes. Remove from the water, and peel away the husk. Crush the peanuts with a pestle or grinder. Transfer the crushed peanuts to a cup.

Heat the soymilk in a saucepan. When hot, pour the soymilk into the cup with the peanuts.

Take one cup twice a day, morning and evening.

Dandelion Wine

👍👍 ✌️

> **12 dandelion leaves (approximately 3 tablespoons or 45 grams),**
> **washed and chopped**
> **2 cups (500 milliliters) rice wine, or sake**

Place the dandelion leaves in a bottle with the rice wine. Seal the bottle and leave to macerate for at least 15 days.

Take 2 teaspoons two times a day.

Abdominal Pains Following Childbirth

In the days and weeks following birth, the uterus slowly contracts to its pre-conception shape and size. The uterine contractions can cause mild to moderate cramping, and consequent pains in the belly area.

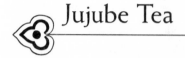

Jujube Tea

5 jujube (Chinese dates)
1 tablespoon (15 grams) minced fresh ginger
1 tablespoon (15 grams) brown sugar
2 cups (500 milliliters) water

In a small saucepan, add all the dry ingredients to the water. Boil over a low flame for 15 minutes.
Consume warm.

SEXUAL PROBLEMS

In the course of our research, we found many and varied remedies for common male sexual problems, such as premature ejaculation, seminal emission, and impotence. However, we found nothing for female problems. When we asked about remedies we were merely met by amused bewilderment. "What female sexual problems? There aren't any, are there?"

We explained that we meant frigidity. This led to even greater bewilderment. "That's a love problem. What remedies can there be for love?"

In China, what matters most is the capacity to bear offspring, not to enjoy the intimacy that leads to conception. As a result, remedies have evolved to cure menstrual problems and those directly related to childbearing. In regard to the male, any weakness in the sperm or in the ability to copulate is considered a threat to successful continuation of the family lineage, and thus merits a cure.

Although a few sexual problems, such as impotence for example, may have an anatomical base, most are entirely psychological in origin. Premature ejaculation and nonphysiological impotence may be due to stress, anxiety, or physical exhaustion. Several methods exist to cure these.

Both impotence and premature ejaculation may be cured by meditation, a positive attitude, qi gong exercise, practical techniques, and a correct diet. Frequent seminal emission, by which Chinese doctors mean a nocturnal emission that spontaneously occurs twice a week or more when you are not having sex, may be corrected through diet. Impotence that is not physiological can also disappear if one overcomes anxiety, has fallen in love, or happens to be in the company of a beautiful member of the opposite sex.

Meditation

Meditation serves to relax. One just sits, preferably in a cross-legged position, and breathes slowly with eyes closed. Concentrate on breathing. Ignore thoughts that may pass through the mind. Meditate every day at the same time before going to bed.

Another meditation technique is to concentrate on a suitable object, concept, or theme. The "seed" that you meditate upon depends on the problem you are trying to cure. If it is premature ejaculation, meditate on sex either beforehand or during the act itself. You need to render sex as impersonal as possible. You can meditate on the cosmic principal of Yin (female) and Yang (male), or on the significance of this Yin-Yang union in all things. You may objectify your own lovemaking by meditating upon the union of Tantric deities, as Tibetan and Mongolian Buddhists do in China. To do this, imagine yourself as one of the deities and see your partner as the embodiment of that deity's female aspect. Or, before making love, you may visualize this tantric act of cosmic sexual union.

If on the other hand you suffer from impotence that is due to stress or anxiety, your seed for meditation needs to be erotically stimulating, and at the same time as relaxing as possible. Close your eyes, breathe slowly and deeply, and meditate on the healthy joys of sex. Fantasize during meditation. Allow the mind to hold steady on whatever sexual theme arouses you—under no circumstances, however, must you stimulate yourself physically. This exercise is entirely mental. Any physical involvement during the meditative fantasy would defeat the purpose of the exercise. Stay detached—fantasize and observe with relaxed detachment.

Qi Gong Exercises

In order to overcome sexual problems, one must learn to control and come to terms with one's physical energy, including the sexual aspect of it. Qi gong is one of the most effective means of doing this. Qi gong calms the nerves, distracts a worried or wayward mind, and builds strength and energy.

You can circulate energy inside the body by means of nei dan qi gong, or internal circulation (see page 245). You may also learn to observe and to control the emotions through meditation and deep breathing, or work off tension through wai dan (external circulation) exercises (see page 248).

If premature ejaculation is the problem, controlled deep abdominal breathing during lovemaking can help. When the urge to ejaculate becomes overpowering, simply hold your breath. This will distract momentarily from the excitement at hand and will reestablish some measure of control over the emotions.

For preventive therapy, qi gong has the following exercise to offer. Lie down in bed with a thick pillow behind your neck. Concentrate on the dan tian, the center of energy four inches below your navel, and massage your abdominal area. Place your left palm flat against your navel and your right palm over your left hand. Beginning with an upward movement from left to right, make thirty-six circles around your navel with your palms. Now place your right palm against your abdomen with the left hand over the top. Make thirty-six circles in the opposite direction.

The second stage of the exercise is to place your palms flat against your abdomen with your thumbs touching the rib cage, your fingers pointing toward one another about six inches apart. Rub your fingers vertically down your abdomen to your groin. Reverse the motion and bring your hands back up to your ribs. Repeat this movement thirty-six times at a rate of one stroke per second. On the downward stroke, pressure should be on your thumbs; on the upward stroke, pressure is on your little fingers. Daily practice is said to assure a definite cure against premature ejaculation.

Another technique similar to that just described but not a true qi gong exercise consists of lying on your back and pressing the fingertips of both hands into your belly, about four inches below your navel. This technique is said to cure premature ejaculation. The technique should be practiced five minutes before getting up in the morning, and again at night before going to sleep. The exercise also serves to massage the liver and kidneys.

There is one more technique that we feel we should mention. It comes from a rural area in central China. While we do not know if any readers will take it seriously, the nature of human sexual curiosity is such that this might turn out to be the most often tried remedy in the whole book.

Take one piece of dry ginger. Peel and then roast it. Place it warm inside your anus before making love. It is said to raise the Yang most wonderfully.

Correct Diet

To prevent or allay sexual problems, one should refrain from smoking, drinking too much caffeine, taking alcohol or drugs, consuming saturated fats, or eating sugars and candies that only provide a rush of energy and no stamina. One should, on the other hand, consume protein and carbohydrates—a common source is walnuts. You can roast walnut meats in a dry frying pan or wok over a low flame for 3 minutes, then grind them into a coarse powder with a pestle or grinder. Eat the walnuts for ten days before going to bed. No quantities have been specified because you can eat as much as you like. You can also eat 10 raw walnuts every day for one month.

One of many Chinese men's favorite source of protein when it comes to treating any form of sexual weakness hearkens back to the dictum that a person can treat a problem in one's own organs by eating the corresponding organ of an animal. We shall refrain, however, from describing the various recipes that involve the sexual apparati of dogs, deer, and bulls. More traditional foods are used in many remedies. It is these, therefore, that we shall limit ourselves to describing.

Kidney and Walnuts

4 cups (1 liter) water
2 pork kidneys, washed and shredded
10 walnut meats, chopped
2 garlic cloves, peeled and minced
3 teaspoons (15 grams) sliced fresh ginger
Salt to taste

In a medium saucepan, bring the water to a boil. Add the kidneys, walnuts, garlic, and ginger to the water. Cover and boil over a medium flame for 30 minutes.

Remove from heat. Drain, and discard the water. Add salt according to taste.

To be eaten twice a week as part of a meal.

Cucumber and Sugar

1 medium cucumber, chopped fine
1 tablespoon (15 grams) white sugar

Mix the cucumber with the sugar. Let the mixture sit for 2 hours.
Strain the cucumbers and discard the juice before eating.

Pork with Lotus Seed

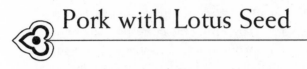

2 tablespoons (30 grams) lotus seeds
Water for soaking
6 cups (1.5 liters) water
½ pound (250 grams) lean pork, cut into 1-inch cubes
2 teaspoons (10 grams) fresh ginger, sliced
2 garlic cloves, peeled and minced
Salt to taste

Soak the lotus seed overnight in 1 cup (250 milliliters) of water. Drain.
In a large soup kettle, bring 6 cups (1.5 liters) of water to a boil. Add the diced pork, lotus seeds, and ginger and garlic. Boil over a medium flame for 1 hour, covered. Add salt to taste. Drain, discarding the water.
Eat two times a week, as part of a meal.

Eggs, Lotus Seed, and Mushroom Soup

1 tablespoon (15 grams) wood-ear mushrooms
Water for soaking
4 cups (1 liter) water
8 lotus seeds
1 tablespoon (15 grams) taro root, cut into ½-inch cubes
2 eggs
2 teaspoons (10 grams) sugar, white or brown

Soak the mushrooms in hot water for 1 hour. Drain.
Bring the remaining 4 cups (1 liter) of water to a boil in a medium saucepan. Add the lotus seeds, taro root, and mushrooms to the boiling water. Boil over a medium flame for 30 minutes.
Break the eggs and allow them to drop gently into the soup. Add the sugar. After 5 minutes, remove from heat.
Take the soup hot or warm, at least once a week.

In China, the preferred meat for sexual problems is mutton. The following are two common mutton recipes.

178

Mutton Stew

2 tablespoons (30 milliliters) cooking oil
$^1/_2$ pound (250 grams) mutton, cut into 1-inch cubes
6 cups (1.5 liters) water
$^1/_4$ cup (60 milliliters) soy sauce
1 teaspoon (5 milliliters) cooking wine
1 scant teaspoon (4 grams) sugar
2 teaspoons (10 grams) chopped scallion
1 teaspoon (3 grams) sliced fresh ginger
Pinch of anise seed
$^1/_4$ cup potato (50 grams), cut into 1-inch cubes
$^1/_4$ cup carrot (50 grams), cut into 1-inch cubes

Heat the oil in a wok or frying pan. Add the mutton and stir-fry for 5 minutes.

Transfer the mutton to a soup kettle. Add the water and all remaining ingredients except the potato and carrot. Bring to a boil, then simmer, covered, on a low flame for 1 hour.

Add the potato and carrot. Simmer for another 20 minutes. Remove from heat.

Eat once a day as part of a meal, at least two times a week.

Stir-fried Mutton

2 tablespoons (30 milliliters) cooking oil
1 pound (500 grams) mutton, thinly sliced
$^1/_2$ cup (100 grams) scallion, sliced
2 teaspoons (10 grams) chopped ginger
5 tablespoons (75 milliliters) soy sauce
2 tablespoons (30 milliliters) cooking wine
2 tablespoons (30 milliliters) sesame oil

Set a wok or frying pan over high heat. Add cooking oil. When the oil is hot, drop in the mutton, scallion, and ginger. Stir-fry for 1 minute. Add the soy sauce and wine. Continue to stir-fry for 5 minutes, until the color of the meat changes.

Add the sesame oil. Stir. Remove from heat and transfer to a plate for serving.

To be eaten at least twice a week.

Centipede and Licorice

Other dietary suggestions for male sexual deficiencies include seafood (shrimp in particular), dog meat, and centipede. Judging by the quantity of dried centipede for sale in Chinese apothecaries, the latter is quite a popular remedy.

30 dried centipedes (you can purchase centipedes from Chinese pharmacies)
1 teaspoon (5 grams) licorice
¹/₂ teaspoon (2.5 grams) anise seed

Place the centipedes, licorice, and anise seed in a mortar. Using a pestle, crush them into a fine powder.

Take ¹/₂ teaspoon (2.5 grams) of the powder at a time, twice a day, morning and evening.

Finally, perhaps the most important antidote to a sexual problem is to live one's sexuality with joy and freedom from guilt or anxiety. A positive attitude lets us take life more lightly than many people are wont.

SMOKING DEPENDENCY

Stopping smoking is, first of all, a matter of will. One must really want to stop smoking in order to continue with a full and healthy life. The strategy, once the decision has been made, is to steer away from circumstances that create the urge or that perhaps simply remind one of the old habit—if, for example, you are in the habit of smoking an after-dinner cigarette with coffee, give up the coffee.

Flush out the nicotine that remains in the body. Drink plenty of water and fresh fruit juices. Fast. After the fast, eat fresh fruit and vegetables for at least ten days. Stay active with qi gong breathing exercises.

Control your urge to smoke for two weeks, and try the following Chinese remedy during that period.

Fresh Daikon Juice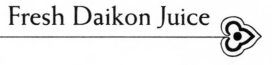

👍👍👍 ✋

1 fresh daikon, grated
1 tablespoon (15 grams) sugar, white or brown

Using a thin towel, squeeze the daikon to extract the juice. Pour the juice into a glass, add the sugar, and stir well. Consume before breakfast.

Daikon juice should be drunk every morning for two weeks. If, at the end of the two weeks, you try to smoke, you supposedly will find cigarettes both tasteless and dissatisfying.

STOMACHACHE

According to traditional Chinese medicine, stomachache is due to careless eating habits, unhappiness, weak Yang, or too much cold. Refer to chapter 3 for information about how to avoid these pitfalls.

When you are suffering from stomachache, avoid taking chili (red pepper), garlic, vinegar, wine or alcohol, strong tea or coffee, bananas, papaya, and cabbage. The following remedies should also come in useful.

Ginger and Sugar Decoction

👍👍👍 ✋

Brown sugar dispels cold and benefits the blood. Ginger warms the stomach. For a more powerful warming effect, use dried ginger.

2 teaspoons (10 grams) fresh or dried ginger
6 tablespoons (90 grams) brown sugar
1¹/₂ cups (375 milliliters) water

Boil the ingredients in a terra-cotta pot or in a small saucepan for ten minutes. Drink hot or warm once a day, until the stomachache goes away.

Ginger and Licorice Decoction

1 stick licorice
$\frac{1}{2}$ tuber of dry ginger
1 cup (250 milliliters) water

Using a pestle or grinder, crush the licorice and ginger.

Place the licorice and ginger in a terra-cotta pot or small saucepan with water. Bring to a boil, then simmer, covered, over low heat for 10 minutes.

Drink warm.

Ginger and Black Pepper Broth

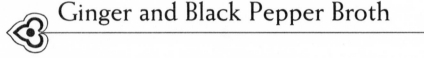

The warming effect of dried ginger may be increased by adding black pepper.

2 teaspoons (10 grams) dried ginger
10 black peppercorns
1 cup (250 milliliters) water

Using a pestle or grinder, crush the ginger and peppercorns into a fine powder. Place the powder in a cup.

Bring the water to a boil. Pour the water into the cup with the powder.

Stir the broth well. Drink hot once a day.

Ginger and Milk with Honey

2 tablespoons (30 grams) grated fresh ginger
1 cup (250 milliliters) milk
1 teaspoon (5 milliliters) honey

Using a thin cotton towel, squeeze the ginger to extract the juice.

Warm the milk in a small saucepan. When the milk is hot, but before it boils, add the ginger juice. Heat for another minute or so.

Remove from heat, transfer to a cup, and stir in the honey.

Drink warm before bed.

Ginger Tripe

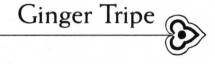

According to the theory that one strengthens the organs of one's body by eating the corresponding animal organ, one can treat stomachache by consuming tripe. Besides being a remedy for chronic stomachache, weakness of the stomach, and general debility, tripe also nourishes qi.

3¹/₂–7 ounces (100–200 grams) pork or other animal tripe
1 cup (250 milliliters) vinegar
2 tablespoons (30 grams) sliced fresh ginger
10 black peppercorns
Water for steaming

Wash the tripe in vinegar. Cut the tripe into strips and place in a ceramic bowl or steaming dish (see page 66).

Add the ginger and pepper to the tripe. Using a pan deep enough to fit your steamer, bring water to a boil. Place the staemer in the pan, cover, and steam for 45 minutes.

Include this dish as part of your lunch and dinner for as long as your stomachache bothers you. Gradually decrease portion size until you are ready to stop the cure altogether.

Cinnamon Tea

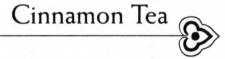

1 cup (250 milliliters) water
1 teaspoon (5 grams) cinnamon powder

In a small saucepan, bring the water to a boil.

Pour the hot water into a cup. Dissolve the cinnamon in the water. Let sit for 10 minutes.

Drink warm as often as you like.

Potato Juice and Honey

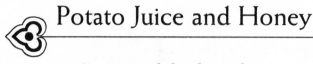

1 potato, peeled and grated
1 teaspoon (5 milliliters) honey

Using a thin cotton towel, squeeze the potato to extract the juice.
Transfer the juice to a cup. Add honey and stir.

Take every morning on an empty stomach for twenty days.

Peanuts with Milk and Honey

This nightcap is taken primarily to relieve stomachache; it can also be used as a treatment for gastritis and gastric ulcers.

4 tablespoons (60 grams) raw peanuts
Water for soaking
1 cup (250 milliliters) milk
2 tablespoons (30 milliliters) honey

Soak the peanuts in hot water for 1 hour. Drain, then grind the peanuts into a pulp using a stone grinder or a mortar and pestle.

In a small saucepan, bring the milk to a boil. When the milk begins to rise, add the ground peanuts. Allow the milk to begin rising for a second time, then remove at once from the flame. Allow the milk to cool for 5 minutes before adding honey.

Take this drink as a nightcap, just prior to going to bed.

WHOOPING COUGH (PERTUSSIS)

Whooping cough is a bacterial infection characterized by extremely troublesome symptoms that give the disease its name. In fact, whooping cough manifests as sudden attacks of intensive coughing followed by a labored inspiration or "whoop" and then by the production of catarrh and by vomiting. The symptoms are so persistent that children cannot eat or sleep because of them. Although modern medicine is to be preferred to traditional rural remedies for curing the ailment, you might wish to try the following remedies to soothe the cough and the catarrh and to strengthen a weakened patient.

Garlic and Sugar

This recipe provides some relief against coughing and the production of catarrh during the first week to ten days of whooping cough. After that, the coughing becomes more intense and requires stronger remedies.

¹/₂ head garlic, peeled and crushed
1 tablespoon (15 grams) brown sugar
1 cup (250 milliliters) water
Water for steaming

Mix the garlic and sugar well. Place the mixture in a ceramic bowl and add 1 cup (250 milliliters) of water. Place the bowl in a steaming dish (see page 66). Using a pan deep enough to fit your steamer, bring water to a boil. Place the steamer in the pan, cover, and steam for 20 minutes.

After steaming, siphon off the solid residue and divide the liquid into three parts. Drink each portion at five-hour intervals.

Chicken Gall Bladder with Sugar

When, after the first ten days of pertussis, coughing becomes more intense and more stubborn, this recipe can help.

1 chicken gall bladder
4 tablespoons (60 grams) sugar, white or brown
¹/₂ cup (125 milliliters) water
Water for steaming

Place the gallbladder in a ceramic bowl together with the sugar and water. Place the bowl in a steaming dish (see page 66).

Using a pan deep enough to fit your steamer, bring water to a boil. Place the steamer in the pan, cover, and steam for 20 minutes.

To be eaten twice a day for five days.

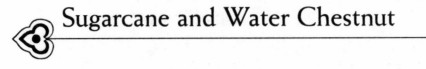

Sugarcane and Water Chestnut

Besides the actual cough, other symptoms of pertussis are vomiting, a high temperature, thirst, and weakness. The following is a remedy for thirst and a high temperature.

> 1 cup (250 milliliters) water
> ½ cup (100 grams) sugarcane, peeled and cut into small pieces
> ½ cup (100 grams) water chestnuts, peeled and cut into small pieces

In a small saucepan, bring the water to a boil. Add the sugarcane and water chestnut. Simmer on a low flame, covered, for 15 minutes.

To be taken as often as desired. All the ingredients should be eaten.

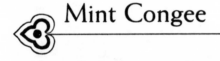

Mint Congee

This remedy is also for thirst and a high temperature.

> ¼ cup (50 grams) rice
> 2 cups (500 milliliters) water
> 20 to 30 fresh mint leaves
> 1 tablespoons (15 grams) rock sugar

Prepare the rice congee by gently boiling the rice and water in a small saucepan for 20 minutes. When the congee is nearly ready, add the mint and the sugar. Simmer for 2 or 3 minutes more.

To be taken hot or warm, three times a day.

The following three remedies are all for coughing. The first remedy is also a general tonic that helps the body regain its strength.

Carrot and Jujube Decoction

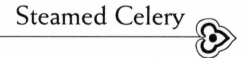

¹/₂ cup (100 grams) carrot, sliced
10 jujube (Chinese dates)
3 cups (750 milliliters) water

Place the carrot in a terra-cotta pot or medium saucepan with the jujube and water. Bring to a boil, then simmer over a low flame, uncovered, for 20 to 30 minutes, until two-thirds of the water has evaporated.

Divide the decoction into ten doses. Take one dose every two hours.

Walnut and Pear Decoction

5 walnuts, chopped
1 pear, finely chopped
3 tablespoons (45 grams) rock sugar
2 cups (500 milliliters) water

Place the walnuts, pear, sugar, and water in a small saucepan. Bring to a boil. Simmer for 20 minutes, covered.

Remove from heat and allow to cool.

Take 1 tablespoon warm three times a day.

Steamed Celery

1 celery stalk, chopped
Salt to taste
Water for steaming

Wash and chop the celery. Add a little salt. Place the celery in a ceramic bowl or steaming diah (see page 66).

Using a pan deep enough to fit your steamer, bring water to a boil. Place the steamer in the pan, cover, and steam for 15 minutes.

Take 1 tablespoon immediately upon waking up and another at around 7 P.M. for three days.

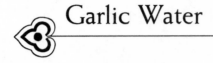

Garlic Water

The final recipe for whooping cough is both a prevention and a cure. As a natural disinfectant and antibiotic, garlic protects when there is a whooping cough epidemic in the area, and soothes coughing and catarrh should your child come down with the illness.

¹/₂ head (60 grams) garlic
2 cups (500 milliliters) tepid water
1 tablespoon (15 grams) brown sugar

Crush the garlic and soak in the water for 10 hours. Remove the garlic solids and add sugar to the water.

A child under the age of five should take 1 to 1¹/₂ teaspoons of the garlic water every two hours. Children over five should take 2 to 3 teaspoons every two hours.

Chapter 6

LONGEVITY BANQUETS

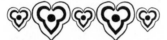

This chapter includes a selection of wholesome Chinese dishes. While most of these recipes have specific curative and preventive functions, all of the dishes can be enjoyed as simply part of a meal.

In China a typical family meal consists of one or two vegetable dishes, a protein dish of tofu, fish, seafood, or meat cooked with vegetables or mushrooms, a bowl of rice, and, perhaps, a soup. The number of dishes depends on the number of people at table. In China all dishes are shared; therefore, the greater the number of people, the greater the variety. When six or eight people eat together, the occasion becomes a veritable banquet. The more people and the more dishes at the banquet, the merrier we feel.

Chinese food is prepared to be enjoyed. Variety is important, as are the food's flavor, its appearance, its smell, and its nutritional value. More important still, however, is the spirit with which we eat it. When we are in the right frame of mind to truly appreciate the food before us, our bodies feel relaxed, our digestive systems are primed, and we benefit tenfold from what we eat.

If, on the other hand, we are tense, worried about weight gain, or feeling guilty about what we are eating, we will not only fail to enjoy, but we shall do more harm to ourselves with this stress than we would by indulging in our "unhealthiest" desires. Such negative emotions impair digestion, waste nutrients, weaken qi, and cause stagnation, creating an environment in which the bodily organs wither and Yin and Yang are thrown out of balance. We then easily fall prey to disease.

189

It is important, therefore, to relax. Invite some good friends over and enjoy a healthy, well-balanced Chinese banquet. Following are some suggestions.

Serving Portions

In China it is believed that eating servings that are too large is unhealthy. Because this book discusses Chinese cuisine for health, the serving portions suggested with the recipes are typical portions in Chinese cuisine. Some books on Chinese cuisine differentiate between Chinese and American servings, suggesting that Americans tend to eat larger amounts of food and that one American serving is roughly equivalent to one and a half Chinese servings. Rather than follow the same kind of format, however, we recommend smaller serving sizes, which we believe are healthier and reflective of Chinese culinary tradition.

A Note on Cooking Methods

Many of the following dishes are prepared in a guo (a wok) or frying pan and entail stir-frying, which does not necessarily require using oil.

Because oil heats to a higher temperature than water, cooking with oil is faster than cooking with water. Oil is recommended for cooking fish and meat dishes; the oils most commonly used in China are peanut oil and vegetable oil. Olive, corn, and canola oil can also be used. Sesame oil, made from roasted seeds, is idea for cold dishes.

In China we believe that animal flesh contains certain toxins that can be eliminated only by thorough cooking, which occurs with the higher temperatures reached when oil is used for stir-frying. If you are positive, however, that your meat or fish is extremely fresh and uncontaminated, you may dispense with using the oil if you wish.

Unlike the thorough cooking required for fish and meat, vegetables when cooked, are prepared so as not to damage heat-sensitive enzymes and vitamins. Stir-frying vegetables serves only to tenderize them and render them more easily digestible. Cooking vegetables with oil is, therefore, not necessary, and you will notice in the recipes that follow that only very short stir-frying times are given for the preparation of vegetable dishes.

SNACKS AND APPETIZERS

Between-meal snacks are not as common in China as they are in the United States. If we feel peckish or bored we usually resort to something like sunflower seeds or watermelon, fresh fruit being a common alternative to seeds. Indeed, it is a Chinese habit to sit and chat over a packet of dried seeds. Anybody who has traveled by train in China will doubtless have noticed the consequences of this habit in terms of litter.

Except for home banquets, appetizers are common in restaurants but not in the home, and usually consist of peanuts or cold cuts of meat, slices of ginger, seaweed, and dried jellyfish. The various appetizers served in Chinese restaurants in America and Europe are not normally eaten in China. Even so, bearing in mind the Western habit of starting a meal with something light, we have included a handful of dishes that can function as either appetizers or snacks.

Tofu and Scallions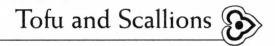

serves 4

Prescribed to alleviate hot- and dry-syndrome diseases, this cold dish replenishes qi and dispels toxic heat. It also counteracts dryness of the throat and mouth and relieves nasal blockage due to a cold.

1 pound (500 grams) tofu, cubed
¹/₂ cup (100 grams) scallions, chopped
2 tablespoons (30 milliliters) sesame oil
2 teaspoons (10 milliliters) lemon juice
1 tablespoon (15 milliliters) soy sauce
¹/₂ teaspoon (2.5 grams) salt

Place the tofu cubes in a bowl, sprinkle with scallions, and season with sesame oil, lemon juice, soy sauce, and salt. Toss lightly.

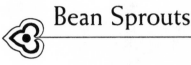

Bean Sprouts

serves 4

Often prescribed as a treatment for chronic dryness in the mouth and throat and for scanty urine, this dish dispels toxic heat and damp syndromes. It also alleviates a sore throat.

> 4 cups (1 liter) water
> 2 cups (400 grams) bean sprouts
> 1 teaspoon (5 milliliters) sesame or olive oil
> 1 teaspoon (5 milliliters) vinegar
> 1 tablespoon (15 milliliters) soy sauce
> ¼ cup (50 grams) scallions, chopped

Bring water to a boil in a medium saucepan. Throw in the bean sprouts and boil for 1 minute.

Remove the bean sprouts, strain, and allow them to cool. Season with oil, vinegar, and soy sauce.

Add the scallions, toss lightly, and serve.

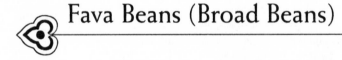

Fava Beans (Broad Beans)

serves 4

Sometimes prescribed as a remedy for indigestion, this dish warms the stomach and the spleen and dispels cold and dampness. Fava beans, also known as broad beans, contain plenty of soluble fiber and are therefore an efficient remedy for constipation. Soluble fiber also lowers cholesterol levels in the blood.

In China, fava beans are usually eaten in summer when people tend to consume large quantities of garlic as a protection against bacteria that develop more easily in the heat. For the Chinese ten or fifteen cloves would be normal. The amount we have suggested for this recipe is 3 tablespoons (45 grams) crushed garlic, less than people would actually use in China. The amount of garlic you use for this dish depends on your fondness for its taste.

> 2 cups (400 grams) fresh fava beans, or 1 cup (200 grams) dried fava
>   beans
> Water for soaking
> 5 cups (1.25 liters) water
> 3 tablespoons (45 grams) crushed garlic
> 2 tablespoons (30 milliliters) sesame or olive oil
> 1 tablespoon (15 milliliters) vinegar
> 2 tablespoons (30 milliliters) soy sauce
> Salt to taste

If using dried beans, soak them overnight and then peel them. If fresh, remove them from their pods.

Bring the water to boil in a large saucepan and add the fava beans. Boil fresh beans over a medium flame for 15 minutes; boil dried beans for 30 minutes.

Remove the beans from the water and strain. Season with crushed garlic, oil, vinegar, and soy sauce, adding salt, if desired, to taste.

Chinese Chicken Salad

serves 4

This dish warms the digestive organs, nourishes qi, stimulates the appetite, and dispels cold- and damp-syndrome diseases.

8 cups (2 liters) water
4 chicken drumsticks
^{1}/2 head iceberg lettuce
1 tablespoon (15 milliliters) sesame oil
1 tablespoon (15 milliliters) hot mustard
^{1}/2 teaspoon (2.5 grams) salt
^{1}/2 teaspoon (2.5 grams) MSG (monosodium glutamate), optional
1 tablespoon (30 grams) ground peanuts (use a mortar and pestle or stone grinder)

In a medium saucepan bring the water to a boil. Add the chicken drumsticks and cook for 30 minutes, or until done. In the meantime, wash, dry, and shred the lettuce.

Remove drumsticks from water and allow to cool. Remove the skin, and debone. Shred the meat into bite-sized pieces.

In a small bowl, combine the sesame oil, hot mustard, salt, and MSG if desired, and mix to make a dressing.

In a large bowl combine the chicken, the shredded lettuce, and the dressing and mix together. Sprinkle the ground peanuts over the salad and serve.

SOUPS

In China soups are generally drunk at the end of the meal rather than at the beginning.[1] We use the term "drunk" rather than "eaten" because soups are typically light, clear broths that serve to wash down the rest of the meal while clearing the mouth and esophagus of strong flavors. Because soups are usually eaten at the beginning of the meal in many Western countries, we have placed them at the beginning of our recipe collection.

Shrimp and Mutton Soup

serves 4 to 6

Mutton is sweet and mild. It nourishes qi and has a warming effect. Shrimp, also sweet and mild, nourish the kidneys and enhance the sexual functions. Garlic is warm and pungent. It dissipates cold and nourishes Yang. This soup is prescribed for kidney deficiencies, aches and pains in the lower body, weakness, cold feet and legs, and urinary problems.

1 teaspoon (5 grams) cornstarch
1 teaspoon (5 milliliters) water
4 ounces (125 grams) fresh shrimp, cleaned,
    peeled, and deveined
2 tablespoons (30 milliliters) cooking oil
2 slices ginger
4 ounces (125 grams) mutton, sliced into fine strips
4 cups (1 liter) water
2 tablespoons (30 grams) crushed garlic
1 scallion, chopped
¹/₂ teaspoon (2.5 grams) salt
¹/₂ teaspoon (2.5 grams) pepper

Mix the cornstarch and the teaspoon of water together in a small bowl and set aside. Finely chop the shrimp.

Heat the cooking oil in a medium saucepan. Drop in the sliced ginger and the mutton, stirring quickly until the mutton changes color (about 3 or 4 minutes), and then add the 4 cups (1 liter) of water. Bring to a boil. Add the garlic, reduce the heat, and simmer over a low flame, uncovered, for 30 minutes.

Add the chopped shrimp and simmer for another 2 minutes. Finally, add the chopped scallion, the cornstarch mixture, and the salt and pepper. Stir until the soup thickens, then remove from the heat. Serve hot.

Mutton and Ginger Soup

serves 4 to 6

This soup strengthens qi and the blood, invigorates the functions of the spleen and stomach, strengthens the body as a whole, and—because of the warming effects of ginger—dissipates internal cold. It also stimulates the appetite. For these many healing properties, this soup is often prescribed to convalescents and to women following childbirth.

12 cups (3 liters) water
1 pound (500 grams) mutton
¹/₂ cup (100 grams) sliced ginger
2 teaspoons (10 milliliters) rice wine
1 scallion, cut into 4 pieces
1 teaspoon (5 grams) salt

Place 4 cups (1 liter) of the water in a soup pot and bring to a boil. Throw in the mutton. After 1 minute, take the meat out of the pot and discard the water.

Cut the mutton into 1-inch or 1¹/₂-inch cubes. Return the cubed mutton to the soup pot along with the remaining 8 cups (2 liters) of water, and the ginger, rice wine, and scallion. Bring to a boil over high heat, then turn down the heat, cover, and let simmer for 1 hour, stirring occasionally, until cooked.

Season with salt when the soup is cooked. Serve hot.

Shrimp and Bean Curd Soup

serves 4 to 6

This soup invigorates the kidneys and stomach. As well, because shrimp strengthens Yang and tofu strengthens Yin, this soup balances both functions.

½ cup (100 grams) packed fresh spinach
1 slice ginger
2 ounces (60 grams) fresh shrimp, cleaned, peeled, and deveined
½ teaspoon (2.5 grams) salt
2 cups (500 milliliters) chicken broth plus 2 cups (500 milliliters) water, or 4 cups (1 liter) vegetable stock
8 ounces (250 grams) tofu, diced
3 tablespoons (45 grams) cornstarch
1 egg, beaten, optional

Wash the spinach and place it in a saucepan. Add the slice of ginger, the shrimp, and the salt. Heat and stir until the spinach has wilted. Add the chicken broth and water (or vegetable broth) and bring to a boil. When boiling, add the diced tofu.

In a small bowl, mix the cornstarch and the cold water. Add the cornstarch mixture to the soup and stir. As soon as the soup begins to boil again, add the beaten egg, if desired. Stir, remove from heat, and serve.

Tofu, Chicken, and Seaweed Soup

serves 4

This low-fat, high-energy dish is suitable for anyone with a weight problem. It also prevents weakness, tendency toward dizziness, and excessive phlegm.

2 ounces (60 grams) chicken breast, cut into ½-inch cubes
Pinch of salt, plus 1 to 2 teaspoons
2 tablespoons (30 milliliters) cooking wine
1 pound (500 grams) tofu, cut into 1-inch cubes
5 cups (1.25 liters) water
2 tablespoons (30 grams) seaweed
2 scallions, chopped

Place the chicken in a medium bowl. Stir in a pinch of salt and the cooking wine.

Place the tofu in a medium saucepan along with the water. Bring to a boil over a high flame. Once the water boils, add the chicken. Return to a boil, then reduce the heat. Cook for 20 minutes over a medium flame.

Stir in the seaweed, chopped scallions, and remaining 1 to 2 teaspoons salt. Turn off the burner. When sufficiently cool, the soup is ready to serve.

Tofu, Pork, and Black Mushroom Soup

serves 4 to 6

This dish warms the stomach, invigorates the functions of digestion, and fortifies qi and the Yin functions of the body. It also alleviates symptoms of dryness, lowers blood pressure, stimulates the appetite, and increases physical energy. It is prescribed to new mothers after childbirth in order to increase lactation and to counteract weakness and dizziness.

5 black mushrooms
Water for soaking
8 ounces (250 grams) lean pork, cut into 1$\frac{1}{2}$-inch cubes
4 slices ginger
4 jujube (Chinese dates)
8 cups (2 liters) water
1 pound (500 grams) tofu, cut into 1$\frac{1}{2}$-inch cubes
1 teaspoon (5 grams) salt

Soak the mushrooms in a bowl of hot water for 1 hour, then drain and slice.

Place the pork, mushrooms, ginger, jujube, and water in a soup pot. Bring to a boil, lower heat, and cook for 1 hour. Add hot water as needed to retain desired soup consistency.

After an hour, add the tofu. Cook for another 20 minutes. Season with salt and serve hot.

Tofu and Seafood Soup

serves 6

Prescribed as part of the dietary regimen for hypertension (high blood pressure) and for impotence, this dish also stimulates the appetite. A soup that cools internal heat and relieves dryness, it invigorates the internal organs of digestion, the spleen, and, in particular, the stomach.

This soup may also be prepared with sole or snapper (cut into ¹/₂-inch cubes before cooking) instead of shrimp.

> **2 shiitake mushrooms**
> **Water for soaking**
> **¹/₄ cup (50 grams) cornstarch**
> **¹/₄ cup (60 milliliters) water**
> **6 cups (1.5 liters) chicken broth, or water**
> **8 ounces (250 grams) tofu, cut into ¹/₂-inch cubes**
> **¹/₂ cup (100 grams) button mushrooms, sliced**
> **¹/₄ cup (50 grams) fresh peas, shelled**
> **8 ounces (250 grams) fresh shrimp, cleaned, peeled, and deveined**
> **2 egg whites, beaten**
> **1–2 teaspoons (5–10 grams) salt**
> **1 teaspoon (5 milliliters) sesame oil**
> **Pepper, to taste**

Place the shiitake mushrooms in a bowl, cover with hot water, and soak for 1 hour. Drain and slice.

In a separate small bowl, whisk together the cornstarch and the ¹/₄ cup (60 milliliters) water and set aside.

Pour the chicken broth (or water) into a soup pot and bring to a boil. Then add the tofu, button and shiitake mushrooms, and peas. Stir for a minute, then add the shrimp.

Reduce heat and simmer over a low flame for 10 minutes. Then slowly add the cornstarch mixture, stirring all the while. Stir in the beaten egg whites and immediately remove from heat.

Season with salt, sesame oil, and pepper to taste. Serve hot.

Tomato Soup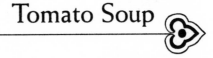

serves 2 to 4

This recipe dispels toxic heat and reinforces the functions of the stomach, stimulating appetite and improving digestion.

2 tablespoons (30 grams) cornstarch
2 tablespoons (30 milliliters) cold water
1 egg
3 cups (750 milliliters) chicken or vegetable broth
2 tablespoons (30 milliliters) soy sauce
1 tablespoon (15 milliliters) vinegar
1/4 teaspoon (1–2 grams) white pepper
2 medium tomatoes, cut into wedges
4 ounces (125 grams) tofu, cut into 1-inch cubes
1 teaspoon (5 milliliters) sesame oil, as garnish
1 tablespoon (15 grams) scallions, chopped, as garnish

In a small bowl, combine the cornstarch and the cold water and mix together thoroughly. Set aside. In another small bowl, beat the egg and set aside.

Place the vinegar and the white pepper in a large serving bowl to be used for the soup. Whisk lightly and set aside.

Pour the broth and the soy sauce into a medium saucepan, stir together, and bring to a boil. When the broth is boiling add the tomato wedges and tofu and return to a boil. Let boil for 5 minutes, then slowly stir in the cornstarch mixture until the soup thickens. Once the soup thickens add the beaten egg, stirring it in using a circular motion, and immediately turn off the heat.

Pour at once into the prepared serving bowl and stir. Garnish with a drizzle of sesame oil and a sprinkle of chopped scallions, and serve.

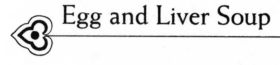

Egg and Liver Soup

serves 2 to 4

This soup is good for the liver and improves eyesight.

2 eggs
1–2 tablespoons (15–30 milliliters) peanut or sesame oil
8 ounces (250 grams) pork liver, thinly sliced
6 green tops of scallions, chopped
1 tablespoon (15 milliliters) cooking wine
2 cups (500 milliliters) water
1 teaspoon (5 grams) salt

Beat the eggs in a small bowl and set aside.

In a medium saucepan, heat the oil. When the oil is hot, add the sliced liver and chopped scallions and stir. Add the tablespoon of cooking wine, stir for 30 seconds more, and add the water. Bring to a boil, lower the heat, and simmer for 15 minutes.

When ready, pour the beaten egg into the soup, stirring it in using a circular motion. Season with salt and serve in a large soup tureen or in individual bowls.

Sweet Corn, Chicken, Mushroom, and Egg Soup

serves 4

Corn is sweet and mild; it lubricates and nourishes the internal organs of digestion. Shiitake mushrooms are sweet and neutral; they nourish the stomach. This dish as a whole strengthens the functions of the stomach, thus stimulating the appetite. It is often prescribed as treatment for urinary problems as well.

4 shiitake mushrooms
Water for soaking
1 chicken breast
2 egg whites
1/2 cup (100 grams) sweet corn
4 cups (1 liter) stock
2 teaspoons (10 milliliters) cooking wine
1 teaspoon (5 grams) salt
1/2 teaspoon (2.5 grams) black pepper

Soak the mushrooms in 1 cup of hot water for 1 hour. Drain. Chop the mushrooms into small pieces and set aside.

Remove the chicken breast from the bone and mince. Set aside.

In a medium bowl, beat the egg whites into a foam. Mix the minced chicken and the cooking wine into the beaten egg whites.

In a medium saucepan add the sweet corn to the stock, bring to a boil, and boil for 10 minutes. Then add the chicken and egg white mixture and the mushrooms to the stock. Lower the heat and let simmer for 5 minutes, stirring occasionally.

Season with salt and pepper and serve.

Vegetable Beef Soup

serves 6

This soup invigorates the spleen and stomach and harmonizes qi. It nourishes the blood and strengthens the bones, joints, and ligaments. It stimulates the appetite, and its energizing properties render it particularly effective for conditions of fatigue, weakness, and convalescence.

**12 cups (3 liters) water
8 ounces (250 grams) beef, cut into 1-inch cubes
$1/2$ cup (100 grams) carrot, chopped into 1-inch pieces
3 slices ginger
$1/2$ cinnamon stick
2 teaspoons (10 milliliters) cooking wine
$1/4$ cup (50 grams) onion, sliced thin lengthwise
$1/2$ cup (100 grams) tomato, chopped into 1-inch pieces
$1/4$ head cabbage, chopped into 1-inch pieces
$1/2$ cup (100 grams) potato, chopped into 1-inch pieces
1–2 teaspoons (5–10 grams) salt
1 tablespoon (15 milliliters) soy sauce**

Bring 4 cups (1 liter) of the water to a boil in a soup pot. Add the beef, return to a boil, and cook for 1 minute. Strain the broth and discard it.

In the same saucepan, add the remaining 8 cups (2 liters) of fresh water to the beef. Throw in the chopped carrot, ginger slices, cinnamon stick, and cooking wine. Bring to a boil, reduce heat, cover, and cook over a low flame for 1 hour.

After 1 hour of cooking, add the onion, tomato, cabbage, and potato. Continue to simmer for another 20 minutes.

Season with salt and soy sauce. Serve hot.

Vegetable Chicken Soup

serves 4 to 6

This soup dissipates heat, relieves water retention, and nourishes the internal organs, invigorating their qi. It is a good remedy for stomachache due to cold syndromes. It is also a treatment for lack of appetite, weakness, convalescence, stubborn coughs, and urinary disorders, and is a favorite among women recovering from childbirth.

This is a convenient recipe that can be made to last for several meals. Also, by eating only a few strips of chicken meat with each bowl of soup, you can keep the chicken as a base. If you prefer, for each meal you can add other vegetables or additional cabbage, or substitute cauliflower for cabbage and cook for 15 more minutes.

1 whole chicken (about 3 pounds or 1½ kilograms)
3 slices ginger
1 cup (200 grams) carrot, cut into 1-inch pieces
½ cup (100 grams) daikon, cut into 1-inch pieces
20 cups (5 liters) water
1 cup (200 grams) Napa cabbage, cut into strips
2 teaspoons (10 grams) salt

Wash the chicken and pat it dry. Cut away the skin and fat.

Place the chicken in a deep saucepan along with the ginger slices, carrot, and daikon. Cover with water and bring to a boil. Reduce heat, cover, and simmer over a low flame for about 1 hour, or until the chicken is cooked.

Add the cabbage and cook for another 15 minutes. Season with salt and remove from heat. Serve warm.

VEGETABLE DISHES

Although few people in China—aside from Buddhist monks—are vegetarians, the Chinese diet does tend to rely more heavily on grains and vegetables than on meats. In 1989 in China only 9 percent of calories were obtained from animal products. The latest available figures show that by 1996 the general improvement of economic conditions and the consequent change in dietary habits led to a 3.8 percent increase in meat consumption. In contrast, in the United States the corresponding figure for calories from animal protein was 34 percent, and in Great Britain it was 35 percent.[2] In China, an ordinary meal in the home only rarely includes more than a few morsels of fish or meat. We reserve meat eating for special occasions, for when we have guests, or for specific health problems.[3] Chinese cuisine, therefore, includes many more recipes for vegetable dishes than for fish, poultry, or other meat dishes. Following are just a few of these.

Sautéed Celery

serves 4

Celery cools the blood and eliminates dampness. It also nourishes and soothes the liver. This dish regulates blood pressure and is prescribed for people who wish to lose weight.

> 2 tablespoons (30 milliliters) oil, or water
> 5 garlic cloves, peeled and crushed
> 2 cups (400 grams) celery, stalk only, cut into 1-inch pieces
> 1 tablespoon (15 milliliters) soy sauce
> Salt and pepper to taste

In a wok or frying pan, heat the oil or water. Drop in the crushed garlic, then throw in the celery. Stir well.

Add the soy sauce and a little salt and pepper, as desired. Stir again, and cover the pan. Cook over a medium flame for 20 to 25 seconds.

Remove from heat and serve.

Mustard Celery

serves 4

Celery cools the blood, eliminates dampness from the body, nourishes and soothes the liver, and lowers high blood pressure. This dish is prescribed for people who wish to lose weight and sometimes—because of the rising effect of the mustard—as a remedy for headache.

1 tablespoon (15 grams) dry mustard
³/₄ tablespoon (11 milliliters) warm water
4¹/₂ cups (1,125 milliliters) water
¹/₄ teaspoon (1–2 grams) sugar
¹/₂ tablespoon (7 grams) cornstarch
Pinch of salt, or to taste
1 cup (200 grams) celery, cut into 1¹/₂-inch pieces

Place the dry mustard in a small bowl and add the ³/₄ tablespoon (11 milliliters) of warm water. Mix together to form a paste and let stand for 10 minutes.

Pour ¹/₂ cup (125 milliliters) water into a small saucepan, along with the sugar, cornstarch, and a pinch of salt. Mix together and bring to a boil, stirring well until the mixture thickens. Stir in the mustard paste, remove from heat, and set aside.

Place the remaining 4 cups (1 liter) water in a medium saucepan and bring to a boil. When boiling, throw in the celery. After 30 seconds, remove from the heat and drain.

Place the celery in a serving dish, cover with the mustard sauce, mix thoroughly to coat, and serve.

Spinach with Celery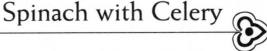

serves 4

This dish prevents high blood pressure, dizziness, palpitations, tinnitus, constipation, and liver problems. Caution: Because spinach contains oxalic acid it should not be eaten with tofu, which contains calcium. When oxalic acid and calcium are mixed, they react to form an indigestible compound.

1 cup (200 grams) packed fresh spinach
3^1/$_2$ cups (875 milliliters) water
1 cup (200 grams) celery, chopped
2 teaspoons (10 milliliters) sesame oil
1 tablespoon (15 milliliters) soy sauce
1 teaspoon (5 milliliters) vinegar

Wash the spinach thoroughly. Place it in a small saucepan with ^{1}/$_2$ cup (125 milliliters) of water and bring to a boil. Reduce the heat and simmer for 5 minutes.

Place the remaining 3 cups of water in a separate medium saucepan, add the celery, and bring to a boil. Reduce heat and simmer for 5 minutes. When cooked, strain the spinach and the celery and place them together in a serving bowl.

In a small bowl whisk together the sesame oil, soy sauce, and vinegar to make a dressing. Pour over the spinach and celery and toss lightly to combine. Serve hot.

Sautéed Asparagus

serves 4

Asparagus dissipates toxic heat from the body, lubricates dryness, acts as a diuretic, lowers blood pressure, and benefits qi, blood circulation, and the heart.

2 tablespoons (30 milliliters) oil, or water
4 garlic cloves, peeled and crushed
2 cups (400 grams) asparagus, cut into 1^1/$_2$-inch pieces
2 tablespoons (30 milliliters) soy sauce
3 tablespoons (45 milliliters) water
Salt and pepper to taste

Heat a wok or frying pan with the oil (or water). When the oil is hot, drop in the crushed garlic and stir. Lower the flame to medium. Add the asparagus and stir. Add the soy sauce and stir-fry for 30 seconds.

Add the 3 tablespoons of water, cover the pan, and simmer for 30 more seconds.

Salt and pepper to taste and stir well. Remove from heat and serve.

Lohan Jai, "Buddha's Delight"

Lohan, or Arhat to use the Sanskrit name, are the Buddha's principle disciples. The name of this dish may thus be translated as "vegetarian dish (jai) of Buddha's disciples." It is considered one of the tastiest and most nutritious dishes for vegetarians.

Lohan jai's properties strengthen qi, dispel dampness, and warm the stomach. In China this dish is often eaten as part of a therapeutic regimen for lowering high blood pressure. It is a favorite among people who feel weak or tired, and among the elderly.

6 shiitake mushrooms
¹/₂ ounce (15 grams) wood-ear mushrooms
¹/₂ ounce (15 grams) dry lily flowers
³/₄ ounce (20 grams) tofu
Water for soaking
2 tablespoons (30 milliliters) oil, or water
5 garlic cloves, peeled and crushed
¹/₂ cup (100 grams) peeled potatoes, thinly sliced
2 teaspoons (10 milliliters) cooking wine
2 tablespoons (30 milliliters) soy sauce
10 ounces (300 grams) gluten, braised
Salt to taste

Place the shiitake mushroons, wood-ear mushrooms, dry lily flowers, and tofu in separate bowls. Cover each ingredient with hot water and soak until they are soft. If you are in a hurry, 45 minutes is the bare minimum for palatability. (In China, most cooks soak these overnight.)

When they are soft, strain the shiitake mushroons and reserve the soaking water, setting it aside. Drain all other soaked ingredients. Slice the shiitake and wood-ear mushrooms. Cut the soaked tofu into 1-inch-long (about 2-centimeter-long) segments.

Heat the oil (or water) in a wok or frying pan. Add the crushed garlic and stir-fry for 5 seconds. Add the sliced potato, the shiitake and wood-ear mushrooms, the lily flowers, and the tofu and stir. Add the cooking wine and the soy sauce and stir thoroughly.

Add about ¹/₄ cup (60 milliliters) of the water in which you soaked the shiitake mushrooms. Cover the wok and allow to simmer for 5 minutes, stirring occasionally and adding a little water if needed.

After 5 minutes, add the braised gluten. Stir well. Cover the pan again and simmer for another 5 minutes.

Add salt to taste, remove from heat, and serve.

Spicy Eggplant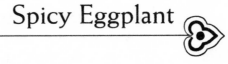

serves 2 to 3

This dish stimulates the stomach and the spleen as well as the functions of digestion, and thus improves the appetite.

1½ tablespoons (23 grams) cornstarch
2 tablespoons (30 milliliters) water
2 tablespoons (30 milliliters) cooking oil, or water
2 cups (400 grams) eggplant, peeled and cut into 2-inch-long (4-centimeter-long) strips
1 teaspoon (5 milliliters) sesame oil
1 scallion, chopped
2 teaspoons (10 grams) grated ginger
3 garlic cloves, peeled and crushed
3 teaspoons (15 grams) chili paste
2 teaspoons (10 grams) black bean paste
2 teaspoons (10 milliliters) cooking wine
2 tablespoons (30 milliliters) soy sauce
1 teaspoon (5 grams) sugar
1 teaspoon (5 milliliters) vinegar
Salt to taste

Blend the cornstarch with 2 tablespoons (30 milliliters) of water in a cup or small bowl and set aside.

Heat the cooking oil, or water if you prefer, in a wok or frying pan. Add the eggplant and stir-fry for 5 minutes until it is soft (10 minutes if you are using water). Transfer to a dish and set aside.

Place the sesame oil in the wok or frying pan and reheat the pan. Add the scallion, ginger, garlic, and chili paste. Stir for a few seconds, until the ingredients give off their aroma, then add the black bean paste, cooking wine, soy sauce, sugar, and vinegar. Stir quickly, then add the eggplant together with the cornstarch, stirring until thoroughly combined. Sprinkle with salt to taste.

Turn off the heat. Transfer to a serving bowl or platter and serve.

Multiflavored Eggplant

This eggplant dish strengthens qi, invigorates circulation of blood, and dispels toxic heat and evil wind syndromes. It is suitable for people with high blood pressure and also provides relief for constipation and hemorrhoids. As well, the generous amount of garlic acts as an antibiotic, curing stomach problems and sore throat.

> **2 cups (400 grams) eggplant, peeled and cut into strips**
> **Water for steaming**
> **1 head garlic, cloves peeled and crushed**
> **1 scallion, chopped**
> **1 tablespoon chopped cilantro**
> **2 tablespoons (30 milliliters) soy sauce**
> **1 teaspoon (5 grams) sugar, optional**
> **1 tablespoon (15 milliliters) vinegar**
> **1 teaspoon (5 milliliters) sesame oil**
> **Salt and pepper to taste**

Place the eggplant in a ceramic bowl, then put the bowl inside a steaming dish (see page 66).

Using a pan deep enough to fit your steamer, bring water to a boil. Place the steamer inside the pan, cover, and steam for 20 minutes.

In a small bowl, mix together the crushed garlic, chopped scallion, and cilantro. Stir in the soy sauce, sugar (if desired), vinegar, sesame oil, and a little salt and pepper to taste.

Remove the eggplant from the steamer. Transfer to a serving dish and pour the garlic sauce over it. Serve hot.

Spinach and Bean Sprouts

A dish that nourishes qi and the blood and counteracts dryness and toxic heat syndromes, it is prescribed for headaches, dizziness, high blood pressure, and constipation.

> **½ cup (100 grams) packed fresh spinach**
> **½ cup (100 grams) bean sprouts**
> **3 tablespoons (45 milliliters) water**
> **3 garlic cloves, peeled and crushed**
> **3 tablespoons (45 milliliters) water**
> **Salt to taste**

Wash and drain the spinach and the bean sprouts.

Heat the water in a wok or frying pan. When the water begins to boil, add the garlic, followed immediately by the spinach and the bean sprouts, and stir. Add salt to taste.

Simmer over medium heat for 5 minutes, until just cooked. Remove from heat and serve.

Steamed Tofu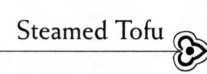

serves 4

This dish removes pathogenic heat from the lungs and dissolves catarrh. It both tones and nourishes the internal organs of digestion, particularly the spleen and the stomach. It also reinforces Yin essence, and relieves dryness.

Steamed tofu is often prescribed for people who are overweight and for those who suffer from indigestion. Because it dissolves catarrh, this dish is frequently taken as a remedy for nasal blockage, coughs, and heavy colds.

1 pound (500 grams) tofu
Water for steaming
2 tablespoons (30 grams) chopped cilantro
2 tablespoons (30 milliliters) lemon juice
3 tablespoons (45 milliliters) soy sauce
1 tablespoon (15 milliliters) sesame oil
Salt to taste
Chili spice, optional

Place the tofu in a steaming dish (see page 66). Using a pan deep enough to fit your steamer, bring water to a boil. Place the steamer inside the pan, cover, and steam for 20 minutes.

When it is finished, remove the tofu from the steamer and cut into 1 1/2-inch cubes.

To make a sauce, mix the cilantro with the lemon juice, soy sauce, sesame oil, a little salt, and chili spice if you like it spicy.

Pour the sauce over the tofu. Mix well and serve.

Tofu with Mushrooms

serves 2

Because of tofu's cooling effect, this dish dispels pathogenic heat from the stomach and the lungs. It also nourishes Yin essence. It is often prescribed to people with diabetes.

5 shiitake mushrooms
2 tablespoons (30 grams) wood-ear mushrooms
2 tablespoons (30 grams) dry lily flowers
Water for soaking
2 tablespoons (30 milliliters) oil, or water
4 garlic cloves, peeled and crushed
8 ounces (250 grams) tofu, cut into 1½-inch cubes
2 tablespoons (30 milliliters) soy sauce
Salt and pepper to taste

Put the shiitake mushrooms, the wood-ear mushrooms, and the dry lily flowers in separate bowls, cover each with hot water, and soak for 1 hour. (Soaking them overnight will ensure the perfect consistency, however 1 hour of soaking is sufficient if you are in a hurry.)

When the shiitake mushrooms are soft, strain them, reserving the water in which they were soaked. Set the reserved liquid aside. Drain the wood-ear mushrooms and the lily flowers, discarding their soaking water. Slice all the mushrooms.

Heat the oil (or water, if you prefer) in a wok or frying pan. When hot, add the crushed garlic and the tofu. Stir-fry for 1 minute (4 minutes if you are using water), then add the shiitake and wood-ear mushrooms and the lily flowers.

Stir in the soy sauce, mixing thoroughly. Add ¼ cup (60 milliliters) of the water in which you soaked the shiitake mushrooms. Cover the wok, reduce heat, and let simmer over a low flame for 10 minutes.

Season with salt and pepper to taste. Remove from heat and serve.

BEEF DISHES

Cabbage Beef

serves 4

This dish nourishes the spleen and stomach, alleviates stomachache, builds physical strength and resistance, and stimulates appetite.

1 tablespoon (15 milliliters) cooking wine
1 tablespoon (15 milliliters) soy sauce
Salt and pepper to taste
1 teaspoon (5 grams) sugar, optional
2 ounces (60 grams) beef, sliced into thin, 3-inch-long
    (7-centimeter-long) strips
2 tablespoons (30 milliliters) cooking oil
5 garlic cloves, peeled and crushed
3 slices ginger
2 cups (400 grams) cabbage, sliced into thin, 3-inch-long
    (7-centimeter-long) strips
2 tablespoons (30 milliliters) water

Place the wine, soy sauce, salt and pepper to taste, and sugar (if desired) in a bowl and combine to make a marinade. Add the beef, stir to coat, and let stand for 15 minutes.

When the beef has been marinated, heat 1 tablespoon (15 milliliters) of the oil in a wok or frying pan. Transfer the beef to the wok. Quickly stir-fry until the beef changes color, then remove it from the wok.

Heat the remaining tablespoon of oil in the wok. Add the garlic and the ginger. Stir for a few seconds before adding the cabbage and 2 tablespoons (30 milliliters) of water. Stir-fry for 4 minutes.

Add the beef. Stir briefly, salt to taste, and serve.

Beef with Prickly Pear Cactus

serves 2

Beef is sweet and mild; it nourishes the spleen and the stomach. Prickly pear cactus is cold and bitter; it removes evil heat and heat inflammation. Together these ingredients balance cold and warm within the body. In China it is believed that if this dish is eaten regularly it will banish all problems of the stomach and the digestive organs.

  1 tablespoon (15 milliliters) soy sauce
  4 slices ginger
  1 tablespoon (15 milliliters) cooking wine, optional
  3 ounces (90 grams) beef, sliced into 3-inch-long
     (7-centimeter-long) strips
  1 tablespoon (15 grams) cornstarch
  1 tablespoon (15 milliliters) water
  2 tablespoons (30 milliliters) oil
  2 ounces (60 grams) prickly pear cactus, sliced into
     3-inch-long (7-centimeter-long) strips
  Salt to taste

Combine the soy sauce, cooking wine (if desired) and ginger in a bowl.

Mix the cornstarch and water in a small bowl. Add the beef and marinate for 5 to 10 minutes. Set aside.

Heat the oil in a wok or frying pan. Drop in the beef and stir-fry until the meat changes color. Add the cactus and stir-fry for 2 or 3 minutes.

Add a little salt. Pour in the cornstarch and stir again. Remove from heat and serve.

Onion Beef

serves 2

This dish nourishes qi and the blood, strengthens the bones and ligaments, and stimulates the appetite. Onion and beef also reinforce the functions of the spleen and the stomach.

  1 tablespoon (15 grams) cornstarch
  1 tablespoon (15 milliliters) soy sauce
  1 tablespoon (15 milliliters) cooking wine
  9 ounces (255 grams) beef, sliced into thin, 3-inch-long
     (7-centimeter-long) strips
  3 tablespoons (45 milliliters) cooking oil
  ¼ cup (50 grams) onion, shredded or grated
  Salt to taste

Place the cornstarch, soy sauce, and cooking wine in a medium bowl and mix well. Add the beef strips and mix to coat.

Heat the oil in a wok or frying pan. When the oil is hot, add the beef and the onion and stir-fry for 5 minutes.

Add salt to taste. Remove from heat and serve.

LAMB AND MUTTON DISHES

Mutton, Taro, and Mushroom

serves 2

Mutton strengthens Yang energy. It nourishes the blood, stimulating its circulation, and reinforces the kidneys. This dish is a valid tonic for the whole body and is therefore effective in overcoming debility, exhaustion, and convalescence.

2 tablespoons (30 grams) wood-ear mushrooms
Water for soaking
1 tablespoon (5 grams) cornstarch
2 tablespoons (30 milliliters) cooking wine
1 tablespoon (15 milliliters) soy sauce
Salt to taste
9 ounces (255 grams) mutton or lamb, cut into
    1-inch by 2-inch pieces
3 ounces (90 grams) taro
3 tablespoons (45 milliliters) cooking oil
2 teaspoons (10 grams) chopped onion
3 slices ginger
1 teaspoon (5 milliliters) sesame oil

Place the wood-ear mushrooms in a small bowl, cover with hot water, and soak for 1 hour. When soft, drain the mushrooms and dry them.

Place the cornstarch, cooking wine, soy sauce, and salt in a bowl and mix together. Add the lamb or mutton pieces and stir to coat.

Chop the taro into pieces about the same size as the meat.

Heat 2 tablespoons of the cooking oil in a wok or frying pan. Add the meat and stir-fry for 5 minutes, or until the meat changes color. Remove the meat from the pan and and set aside in a clean dish.

Heat the remaining tablespoon of cooking oil in the wok. Drop in the onion and ginger and stir for a few seconds. Add the taro and wood-ear mushrooms. Stir-fry for 3 minutes, then mix in the meat. Stir well.

Sprinkle the sesame oil over the dish and add a little salt to taste.

Remove from heat and serve.

Garlic Mutton

serves 2

This dish warms the spleen and the kidneys. It reduces swelling and relieves inflammation due to a preponderant Fire element, and is prescribed as a specific remedy for swelling, pain, cold, and numbness in the knees and joints. It also detoxifies and is sometimes prescribed for impotence and chronic nephritis (inflammation of the kidneys).

9 ounces (255 grams) mutton, cut into 1-inch cubes
4 cups (1 liter) water
1 large head garlic, peeled
Salt and pepper to taste

In a medium saucepan, bring the water to a boil. Add the mutton and the garlic, cover, turn the flame to low, and stew for 1¹/₂ hours, or until cooked. (In China meat is considered fully cooked when the tip of a chopstick pushes through with ease.) Add a little hot water occasionally, to keep the stew from drying out.

Add salt and pepper according to your taste.

Mutton and Shrimp Pudding

serves 2

This dish warms and reinforces the kidneys. Often prescribed to alleviate cold syndromes in the lower half of the body, it corrects urinary deficiencies, soothes pains in the waist and knees, decreases the frequency of seminal emissions, and calms chronic kidney inflammations.

1 tablespoon (15 grams) cornstarch
1 tablespoon (15 milliliters) water
5 ounces (155 grams) mutton, finely shredded
1 tablespoon (15 milliliters) cooking oil
2 slices ginger
³/₄ cup (180 milliliters) water, plus more for thinning
2 tablespoons minced garlic
3 ounces (90 grams) fresh shrimp, cleaned, peeled, and deveined
1 tablespoon (15 milliliters) cooking wine
1 tablespoon (15 milliliters) soy sauce
2 scallions, chopped
Salt and pepper to taste

Mix the cornstarch and the tablespoon of water in a small bowl. Dice the shrimp.

Heat the oil in a wok or frying pan. Drop in the mutton and the ginger. Stir for 10 seconds, then add ³/₄ cup (185 milliliters) of water. Allow the water to come to a boil, then add the garlic. Wait another 30 seconds before adding the shrimp, followed by the wine, and finally by the soy sauce.

Cook for 20 minutes. When the water evaporates, add more a little at a time. Be sure not to pour in too much water, though, as the end product should resemble a semicompact pudding more than a soup or a stew.

When the cooking time is almost up, add the chopped scallions and salt and pepper to taste. Finally, add the cornstarch-water mixture and stir. When the dish is compact enough, with a thickness like pudding, remove from heat and serve.

Mutton Stew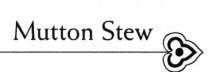

serves 4

Mutton provides strong Yang energy. This dish fortifies the entire body, and the masculine reproductive functions in particular.

> 2 tablespoons (30 milliliters) cooking oil
> 1 pound (500 grams) mutton, cut into 1¹/₂-inch cubes
> ¹/₂ cup (125 milliliters) soy sauce
> 1¹/₂ teaspoons (7 grams) sugar
> 2 teaspoons (10 milliliters) cooking wine
> 6 slices ginger
> 2 tablespoons (30 grams) chopped onion
> 8 cups (2 liters) water
> ¹/₃ teaspoon (2 grams) anise seed
> ¹/₂ cup (100 grams) potato, diced
> 2 carrots, cut into small pieces

Heat the cooking oil in a wok or frying pan and drop the mutton in. Add soy sauce, sugar, and cooking wine, and stir-fry the mutton for about 5 minutes, or until brown.

Pour half of the water into a large soup pot or stove-top casserole dish. Place the ginger slices, onion, and anise seed in the pot with water. Simmer over low heat, covered, for 1¹/₂ hours.

Add the potato and the carrot to the pot, adding water if necessary. Simmer for 20 minutes longer.

Remove from heat and serve in a large tureen or in individual bowls.

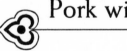

Stir-fried Mutton

serves 2

Like the previous dish, stir-fried mutton also provides strong Yang energy to the body.

1 tablespoon (15 milliliters) cooking oil
¹/₂ pound (250 grams) mutton, thinly sliced
¹/₂ cup (100 grams) scallions, chopped
1 teaspoon (5 grams) chopped ginger
¹/₄ cup (60 milliliters) soy sauce
2 tablespoons (30 milliliters) cooking wine
2 tablespoons (30 milliliters) sesame oil

Set a wok or frying pan over high heat and add the cooking oil. When hot, drop in the mutton, chopped scallions, and ginger and stir-fry.

After 1 minute, add the soy sauce and the wine. Stir-fry for 1 more minute, or until the meat is cooked.

Add the sesame oil and stir, then transfer to a serving plate.

PORK DISHES

Pork with Celery

serves 2

This dish soothes the liver and clears up toxic heat. It also invigorates the functions of the stomach and combats high blood pressure, dehydration, poor appetite, dryness in the mouth, dizziness, and chronic headache.

An alternative to this dish is to use onion in place of celery. Onion warms the internal organs of digestion while celery cools them.

2 ounces (60 grams) lean pork, cut into long shreds
1 tablespoon (15 milliliters) soy sauce
¹/₂ teaspoon (2.5 grams) sugar
2 tablespoons (30 milliliters) cooking oil
3 slices ginger
1 cup (200 grams) celery, cut into 2-inch-long pieces
Pinch of salt

Place the shredded pork in a medium bowl. Add the soy sauce and sugar and mix well. Let marinate for 5 to 10 minutes.

Heat 1 tablespoon of the oil in a wok or frying pan. When heated, drop the ginger into the wok, followed immediately by the marinated pork. Stir for 1 minute, or until pork is cooked to your liking. Transfer temporarily to a separate dish.

Pour the remaining oil into the wok. Reheat and add the celery and a pinch of salt. Stir-fry over high heat for 1 minute, then add the pork. Stir-fry for another 10 seconds. Transfer to a dish and serve hot.

Pork Liver and Bitter Melon

serves 4

In this dish the pork liver and the bitter melon both nourish the blood. Bitter melon detoxifies the blood and cools internal heat syndromes. Eating liver nourishes and strengthens the human liver and cures anemia. Pork Liver and Bitter Melon is known for its ability to alleviate headache and dizziness.

If you dislike the taste of bitter melon, you can blanch the melon for 3 to 4 minutes before frying to remove some of the bitter taste.

1 tablespoon (15 milliliters) soy sauce
1 tablespoon (15 milliliters) cooking wine
$^1/_2$ teaspoon (2.5 grams) sugar
10 ounces (280 grams) pork liver, thinly sliced
$^1/_2$ pound (250 grams) bitter melon (see page 70)
3 tablespoons (45 milliliters) cooking oil
8 garlic cloves, peeled and chopped
1 teaspoon (5 milliliters) sesame oil
Salt to taste

Place the soy sauce, cooking wine, and sugar in a medium bowl and mix together. Add the liver and marinate for 10 minutes.

Cut the bitter melon in half lengthwise. Remove the pulp and the seeds and discard them. Cut the melon into $^1/_4$-inch-thick slices.

Heat 2 tablespoons (30 milliliters) of the oil in a wok or frying pan. Add the sliced liver and half of the garlic. Stir-fry for 4 minutes, then remove and place on a dish.

Place the remaining tablespoon (15 milliliters) of oil in the pan and heat. When the oil is hot, add the remainder of the garlic along with the bitter melon. Stir-fry for 2 minutes, or until evenly cooked. Add the liver and stir for 30 seconds.

Add the sesame oil and salt to taste. Remove from heat and serve.

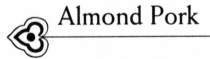

Pied du Porc with Peanuts

serves 2

Because this dish is fairly fatty it is not suitable for everyone. In China it is often taken when one feels weak or fatigued. Pigs' feet provide rich nourishment for qi and the blood. This dish is also prescribed to lactating mothers to stimulate the production of breast milk.

> 1 pig's foot
> ½ cup (100 grams) raw peanuts
> 3 slices ginger
> 1 tablespoon (15 milliliters) cooking wine
> 6 cups (1.5 liters) water

Place all the ingredients in a large saucepan. Bring to a boil, cover the pan, reduce heat to low, and simmer for 1½ hours. Add water as needed. When ready, add salt.

Strain the meat and the peanuts—reserving the water, as you can use it at a later date to prepare a nutritious vegetable soup—and place on a serving dish to serve.

Almond Pork

serves 4

This dish invigorates the functions of the spleen and tones the lungs. It reduces phlegm, relieves coughing, alleviates breathing problems, and is frequently prescribed to people suffering from chronic bronchitis.

> 1 tablespoon (15 grams) almond meats
> Water for soaking
> 1 tablespoon (15 milliliters) cooking oil
> 2 tablespoons (30 grams) sugar
> 1 pound (500 grams) pork, cut into 1-inch pieces
> 1 teaspoon (5 grams) chopped onion
> 1 teaspoon (5 grams) chopped ginger
> 2 tablespoons (30 milliliters) soy sauce
> 1 tablespoon (15 milliliters) cooking wine
> 4 cups (1 liter) water for cooking, plus more as needed

Place the almonds in a small bowl, cover with hot water, and soak for 2 hours or until you can remove the skin with ease.

Heat the oil in a wok or frying pan. Add the sugar and stir-fry for 1½ minutes over medium heat, or until the sugar turns dark red.

Add the pork and stir-fry for 1 minute. Add the onion, ginger, almonds, soy sauce, and wine and stir-fry for 1 more minute. Add the 4 cups of water and continue to cook. (Add more water, a little at a time, if it evaporates too rapidly.) Stew over a low flame for about 1 hour, or until ready. (In China meat is considered done when the tip of a chopstick pushes through with ease.)

Add salt according to taste and serve.

Wood-ear Pork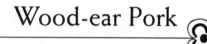

serves 2

This dish alleviates circulation problems and stops bleeding by dispelling pathogenic heat from the blood. In China it is often prescribed to alleviate menstrual pains as well as heavy menstrual bleeding.

¹/₄ cup (50 grams) wood-ear mushrooms
Water for soaking
1 teaspoon (5 milliliters) cooking wine
1 tablespoon (15 milliliters) soy sauce
1 teaspoon (5 grams) cornstarch
4 ounces (115 grams) lean pork, finely sliced
1 tablespoon (15 milliliters) cooking oil
Salt and pepper to taste

Soak the wood-ear mushrooms in hot water for 1 hour, or until soft. Strain and slice.

Combine the wine, soy sauce, pepper, and cornstarch in a medium bowl. Add the pork, stir to coat, and marinate for 10 minutes.

Heat the oil in a wok or frying pan. Drop the pork and the mushrooms into the pan. Stir-fry over high heat for 3 to 4 minutes, or until done.

Add salt and pepper to taste and serve.

Daikon Pork

serves 4

Daikon dispels toxic heat and dissolves phlegm. This dish normalizes the stomach, and thus the functions of digestion. It is an efficient remedy for bloated stomach, indigestion, intestinal gas, and constipation.

1 tablespoon (15 milliliters) cooking oil
2 teaspoons (10 grams) sugar
8 ounces (250 grams) pork, cut into ¼-inch cubes
4 tablespoons (60 milliliters) soy sauce
1 tablespoon (15 milliliters) cooking wine
3 slices ginger
1 tablespoon (15 grams) chopped onion
2 cups (500 milliliters) water
2 cups (400 grams) daikon, cut into ¼-inch cubes
Salt to taste

Heat the oil in a wok or frying pan. Add the sugar and the pork. Stir-fry for 3 to 4 minutes, or until the pork has changed color. Add the soy sauce, wine, ginger, and onion.

Pour the water into the wok to cover the ingredients. Bring to a boil, reduce heat, and simmer over a low flame for 45 minutes. Add the daikon. Continue to cook for 20 more minutes.

Add salt to taste and serve.

Pork with Watermelon

serves 2

This dish dispels heat. It also alleviates thirst, dryness in the throat, headache, and dehydration caused by summer heat or sunstroke.

1 egg white, beaten
1 tablespoon (15 grams) cornstarch
½ teaspoon (2.5 grams) salt, plus a pinch
3½ ounces (100 grams) pork, shredded
½ pound (250 grams) watermelon rind
2 teaspoons (10 milliliters) sesame oil
2 tablespoons (30 milliliters) cooking oil
1 tablespoon (15 milliliters) water

Mix the egg white and the cornstarch in a medium bowl. Add the ½ teaspoon (2.5 grams) of salt.

Place the pork in the bowl with the egg white–cornstarch mixture, stir to coat, and let marinate for 5 minutes.

Wash the watermelon rind thoroughly and remove all but the thick external green shell. Shred the rind. Place the rind in a bowl, sprinkle a pinch of salt over it, then leave to rest for about 5 minutes. After 5 minutes, drain off the water. Add 1 teaspoon (5 milliliters) of sesame oil.

Heat the cooking oil in a wok or frying pan. Add the marinated shredded pork and stir for 3 minutes. Remove, place on a clean plate, and set aside.

Pour the tablespoon (15 milliliters) of water into the pan and place over medium-high heat. Bring the water to a boil, then add the pork and the watermelon rind. Stir for 2 minutes.

Sprinkle the remaining teaspoon (5 milliliters) of sesame oil over the dish, remove from heat, and serve.

CHICKEN DISHES

Jasmine Flower Chicken

serves 2

This dish relaxes the nerves and the nervous system, thus reducing tension. It tones circulation, enriches the blood, and is a good general tonic for combating lack of energy, anemia, and general weakness.

1 tablespoon (15 milliliters) cooking wine
2 egg whites
1 teaspoon (5 grams) cornstarch
1/4 teaspoon (about 1 gram) salt
8 ounces (250 grams) boneless chicken breast, thinly sliced
1 tablespoon (15 milliliters) cooking oil
24 jasmine flowers
Pepper to taste

In a bowl, whisk together the wine, egg whites, cornstarch, and salt. Stir in the chicken and let marinate for 10 minutes.

Heat the oil in a wok or frying pan. Transfer the chicken and the jasmine flowers to the wok. Stir-fry over high heat for 3 minutes, or until cooked. Transfer to a serving dish and sprinkle with a little pepper to taste.

Chestnut with Chicken

serves 4

The strong Yang ingredients in this dish nourish the kidneys and the liver. Because of its strong Yang functions, this dish strengthens male sexuality, combating seminal emission, premature ejaculation, and impotence due to weakness or stress. It also soothes the nerves and combats body pains.

1 cup (200 grams) chestnuts, fresh or dry
Water for soaking
1 tablespoon (15 milliliters) cooking wine
1 tablespoon (15 grams) scallions, chopped
1 tablespoon (15 grams) sugar
2 tablespoons (30 grams) cornstarch
3 cups (750 milliliters) water
2 tablespoons (30 milliliters) cooking oil
1 pound (500 grams) chicken, cut into 1½-inch cubes
4 teaspoons (20 milliliters) soy sauce

Prepare the chestnuts first. If they are dry, soak them in water overnight or until they are soft. If they are fresh, cut a cross in the shell and boil in water for 2 minutes, then peel them. Set aside.

In a medium bowl, mix together the wine, scallions, sugar, cornstarch, and water to make a sauce. Set aside.

Heat the oil in a wok or frying pan. When the oil is hot, place the chicken in the wok, add the soy sauce, and stir-fry for 3 to 4 minutes, or until chicken is golden brown, then add the sauce and the chestnuts. Stir for 1 minute. Add the sauce.

Simmer over a low flame for 30 minutes, or until chicken is cooked, adding a little water if necessary. Remove from heat and serve.

Walnut Chicken

serves 4

This dish invigorates the Yang functions; purifies qi and the blood, stimulating their circulation; and nourishes the kidneys. It is a good remedy for sexual weakness, dizziness, constipation, and lethargy, and prevents premature graying of the hair.

1 egg white
2 teaspoons (10 grams) cornstarch
10 ounces (280 grams) boneless chicken breast, sliced
¼ cup (50 grams) walnut meats
1 tablespoon (15 milliliters) cooking oil
3 shiitake mushrooms, sliced
1 teaspoon (5 grams) finely chopped ginger
1 teaspoon (5 grams) finely chopped scallion
1 teaspoon (5 milliliters) soy sauce
1 teaspoon (5 milliliters) cooking wine
Salt to taste

Place the egg white and cornstarch in a medium bowl and mix well. Add the chicken and stir to coat. Set aside.

Roast the walnuts in a dry wok for 3 minutes, or until golden brown.

Heat the oil in a medium saucepan. When the oil is hot, add the mushrooms, ginger, and scallion. Stir for 30 seconds, then add the chicken. Stir-fry for 2 minutes. Add the soy sauce and the wine. Continue to stir-fry for 3 more minutes.

Drop the walnuts in last and stir-fry for another 30 seconds. Add salt to taste and serve.

Basil Chicken

serves 4

This chicken dish reinforces the functions of the liver and the kidneys and nourishes the skin, rendering it soft and shiny. It also stimulates circulation of the blood and alleviates internal ear problems, including dizziness, tinnitus, and minor hearing problems.

This recipe calls for chicken drumsticks, but chicken breast or other chicken meat may be used if preferred.

1 pound (500 grams) chicken drumsticks
5 garlic cloves, peeled and split lengthwise
1/4 cup (60 milliliters) black sesame oil
5 slices ginger
1/3 cup (90 milliliters) cooking wine
1/4 cup (60 milliliters) soy sauce
1 tablespoon (15 grams) sugar
1/2 cup (100 grams) packed fresh basil leaves

Using a meat cleaver chop each drumstick in half, through the bone. Set the drumstick halves aside.

Heat the sesame oil in a medium saucepan. When the oil is hot, drop in the garlic and ginger and stir for 10 seconds. Then add the chicken. Stir-fry for 2 minutes over high heat. Add the wine, soy sauce, and sugar, reduce the heat, and simmer over a low flame for 20 to 30 minutes, stirring occasionally.

Add the basil leaves. Simmer for 1 more minute and serve.

Pomelo Chicken

serves 4

Grapefruit (pomelo) is sweet, sour, and cold. It eliminates catarrh and strengthens the functions of the stomach, thus aiding digestion. As a whole, this dish invigorates qi. It also reinforces the functions of the spleen, dissolves phlegm, calms coughing, helps digestion, and stimulates the appetite.

1 grapefruit
1 whole chicken (approximately 3 pounds or 1 1/2 kilograms)
1 tablespoon (15 grams) salt
2 white heads of scallion, sliced in half lengthwise
5 slices ginger
1 tablespoon (15 milliliters) cooking wine
4 cups (1 liter) water for steaming

Peel and section the grapefruit and cut each section into three pieces. Clean the chicken inside and out and pat dry.

Place the grapefruit pieces inside the chicken. Rub the salt over the outside of the chicken.

Put the chicken inside a ceramic bowl, together with the scallions, ginger, soy sauce, and wine. Place the bowl with the chicken in a large steaming dish (see page 66).

Bring the water to boil in a large soup pot. When water is boiling, place the steamer in the pot. Cover, turn the heat down to medium, and steam the chicken for 1½ hours. Add hot water to the pot when necessary.

Allow the chicken to cool, then cut it into portions for serving.

Chrysanthemum Chicken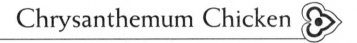

serves 4

This dish nourishes the spleen and liver and improves eyesight. It is good for insomnia, dizziness, and general weakness.

3 egg whites
1 tablespoon (15 milliliters) cooking wine
2 tablespoons (30 grams) cornstarch
½ teaspoon (2.5 grams) salt
1 pound (500 grams) boneless chicken meat, sliced into 2-inch-long pieces
2 tablespoons (30 milliliters) cooking oil
2 teaspoons (10 grams) chopped scallion
2 teaspoons (10 grams) chopped ginger
2 tablespoons (30 grams) dry chrysanthemum flowers
1 teaspoon (5 grams) sugar
1 teaspoon (5 milliliters) sesame oil

Place the egg whites, cooking wine, cornstarch, and salt in a large bowl and mix together. Add the chicken slices and stir to coat.

Heat the cooking oil in a wok or frying pan. Drop in the chopped scallion and ginger. Stir for a few seconds, then add the chicken. Stir-fry for 2 or 3 minutes. Add the chrysanthemum flowers and sugar. Continue to stir-fry for 1 minute.

Remove from heat, place in serving dish, sprinkle with sesame oil, and serve.

DUCK DISHES

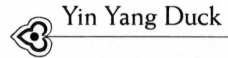

Yin Yang Duck

serves 4

Duck warms the stomach and spleen, reinforces all the vital functions of the body, and invigorates Yang. This duck dish is, therefore, particularly suited to Yang-deficiency syndromes. It also alleviates stomachache and diarrhea caused by low resistance to cold.

1 whole duck (approximately 5 pounds or 2¹/₂ kilograms)
18 cups (4.5 liters) water
5 slices ginger
¹/₄ cup (50 grams) onion, chopped
1 cup (250 milliliters) soy sauce
2 tablespoons (30 milliliters) cooking wine
2 teaspoons (10 grams) salt
2 cinnamon sticks
2 teaspoons (10 grams) anise seed
2 tablespoons (30 grams) sugar

Clean the duck inside and out and pat dry.

Place the duck in a large soup kettle with the water, ginger, and onion. Bring to a boil over high heat. When the water boils, reduce heat to low. Using a spoon, remove the surface foam and discard. Cook for about 20 minutes, until done. The duck is ready when you are able to pass the point of a chopstick through the flesh of the leg.

Turn off the heat. Drain the duck, reserving 2 cups (500 milliliters) of the broth for later use.

Return the duck to the saucepan and add the soy sauce, cooking wine, salt, cinnamon, and anise seed. Add the reserved broth.

Cook over low heat for 15 minutes. Turn the duck over, add the sugar, and cook for another 15 minutes. Near the end of the cooking time, use a spoon to pour the juice over the duck. Transfer the duck to a plate and allow it to cool, then cut and serve individual portions.

Lychee Duck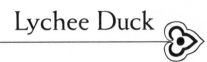

serves 4

This duck dish strengthens the functions of the spleen and nourishes the blood. It also cures anemia, improves the appetite, and invigorates the body as a whole.

This recipe calls for a lotus flower, which is not easy to come by in the United States. If unavailable, a rose—grown without exposure to chemicals or pesticides, of course—may be used.

1 whole duck (approximately 5 pounds or 2¹/₂ kilograms)
1 fresh lotus flower (or rose)
12 cups (3 liters) water
7 ounces (200 grams) lean pork, chopped
1 tablespoon (15 grams) chopped scallion
3 slices ginger
1 tablespoon (15 milliliters) soy sauce
1 tablespoon (15 milliliters) cooking wine
¹/₂ teaspoon (15 grams) salt
Water for steaming
1 cup (200 grams) lychees, fresh or canned

Clean the duck inside and out and pat dry.

Remove the petals from the flower. In a large soup pot, bring the water to boil. Drop the petals into the water and boil for 30 seconds. Remove the petals and set aside, reserving the water for later use.

Mix the pork with the chopped scallion, ginger, soy sauce, wine, and salt in a medium bowl.

Boil the duck in the reserved flower-petal water for 1 minute. Remove the duck and discard the water.

Place the duck in a large steaming dish (see page 66) and spread the pork mixture over it. Using a pot deep enough to fit your steamer, bring the water to a boil. When the water is boiling, place the steamer in the pot. Cover, turn the heat down to medium, and steam the duck for 1 hour, or until cooked. (In China meat is considered fully cooked when the tip of a chopstick can easily pierce the meat.)

Open the steamer, remove the onion and the ginger, and add the lychees and flower petals in their place. Steam for another 15 minutes

Transfer the duck to a plate and allow it to cool, then cut for serving.

EGG DISHES

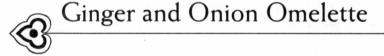

Scrambled Egg with Tomato

serves 2

This dish cools internal heat, nourishes Yin, and stimulates gastric juices, thus improving the appetite. The nerve-relaxing properties of this dish make it a suitable remedy for people suffering from nervous tension, stress, and insomnia.

Because we are not used to sour flavors in China, sugar is generally added to this recipe. Tomato without sugar is deemed too sour. If you like a little sourness, the sugar may be dispensed with.

2 tablespoons (30 milliliters) cooking oil
3 eggs, beaten
3 garlic cloves, peeled and crushed
1 cup (200 grams) diced tomato
1 teaspoon (5 grams) sugar, optional
3 tablespoons (45 milliliters) water
Salt to taste

Heat 1 tablespoon (15 milliliters) of the cooking oil in a wok or frying pan. Add the eggs and scramble for 3 minutes. Remove when ready.

Reheat the wok with the remaining tablespoon of cooking oil (you may use water as an alternative to oil). Throw in the crushed garlic and stir for a few seconds. Add the tomato and, if you wish to use it, the sugar. Stir over medium heat for 2 minutes.

Return the scrambled eggs to the pan and stir well. Add 3 table-spoons (45 milliliters) of water. Cover the wok for 1 minute.

Remove cover, stir, add salt to taste, and transfer to a serving dish.

Ginger and Onion Omelette

serves 2

This omelette dispels pathogenic wind and cold and stimulates the appetite. The ginger and scallion in this dish make it a valid remedy for colds, headaches, coughs, and blocked nasal passages.

3 eggs
1 teaspoon (5 grams) finely minced ginger

4 white heads of scallions, chopped
Pinch of salt, or to taste
1 tablespoon (15 milliliters) cooking oil

Beat the eggs in a medium bowl together with the ginger, scallion, and a pinch of salt.

Heat the oil in a wok or frying pan. When the oil is hot, pour the beaten egg into the pan and cook over a medium flame for 3 minutes. Using a spatula, turn the egg over and cook the top side for 1 minute.

Remove from heat and serve.

SEAFOOD DISHES

Shark

serves 2

Shark cooked with garlic and ginger nourishes the blood and promotes the normal flow of qi; the garlic and ginger in this dish also has a warming effect that dissipates cold and cold-syndrome diseases. This dish invigorates the functions of the stomach. It stimulates the gastric juices, thereby alleviating stomachache and digestive problems, including gas and a bloated abdomen. It also stimulates the appetite. Recent theory asserts that eating shark meat may be a defense against cancer.

1 tablespoon (15 milliliters) cooking oil
1 head of garlic, cloves separated and peeled
3 slices ginger
10 ounces (280 grams) shark, cut into 1-inch cubes
2 teaspoons (10 milliliters) cooking wine
1/2 teaspoon (2.5 grams) sugar, optional
4 tablespoons (60 milliliters) water
1/2 teaspoon (2.5 grams) salt

Heat the oil in a wok or frying pan. When the oil is hot, drop in the garlic cloves and the ginger. Stir for 1 minute, then add the shark meat, cooking wine, and sugar if desired. Stir over medium heat. Add the water, cover the pan, and cook for 2 minutes.

When the fish is cooked, season with salt and serve.

Steamed Trout

serves 2 to 4

Steamed carp is a classic dish in China. In fact, carp is our most common fish. It thrives in the millions of small ponds and rice paddies of eastern China.

Since carp is not common in the United States—and, as a result, it is not the favorite fish of most people—we have based this recipe on another freshwater fish with similar medicinal properties—the trout. Any fish may be prepared in this traditional manner. Steamed salmon steak is one favorite, although salmon is not as lean as carp or trout and has very different medicinal properties than freshwater fish. The most important requirement for this dish is that the fish be fresh.

1 fresh whole trout
4 slices ginger, finely shredded
Water for steaming
2 stalks cilantro
3 scallions, finely chopped
2 tablespoons (30 milliliters) soy sauce
Salt and pepper to taste
1 tablespoon (15 milliliters) sesame or olive oil, optional

Clean the trout and place on a shallow ceramic dish that will fit inside your steamer (see page 66). (If the trout won't fit, cut it in half.) Sprinkle the ginger over the fish.

Using a pan deep enough to fit your steamer, bring water to a boil. Place the steamer in the pan, cover, turn the heat down to medium-low, and steam for 15 minutes.

Turn off the heat and remove the dish from the steamer. Drain off any liquid. Garnish the fish with the cilantro, scallions, and soy sauce. Sprinkle with salt and pepper to taste.

As a finishing touch, you may heat 1 tablespoon (15 milliliters) of sesame or olive oil and sprinkle it over the fish before serving, if desired.

Snapper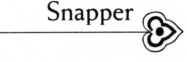

serves 2

Snapper nourishes the spleen and enhances qi. It also counteracts diarrhea.
Although filling, this dish stimulates the appetite.

10 ounces (200 grams) snapper
1 tablespoon (15 milliliters) cooking wine
1 tablespoon (15 milliliters) soy sauce
2 tablespoons (30 milliliters) cooking oil
1 scallion, chopped
2 slices ginger
½ cup (100 grams) taro root, sliced
¼ cup (60 milliliters) water
½ teaspoon (2.5 grams) salt

Cut the snapper into 2-inch-thick slices.

In a medium bowl, mix the cooking wine and soy sauce. Place
the snapper in the bowl and toss to coat. Let it sit for 10 minutes to
marinate.

Heat the oil in a wok or frying pan. Drop in the chopped scallion
and the ginger and stir for a few seconds, then add the snapper and the
taro. Stir for a few more seconds, then add the water. Cover the wok
and let cook for 3 minutes.

Remove from heat. Arrange the snapper on a serving dish. Add salt
and serve.

Ginger Calamari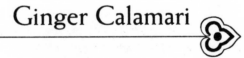

serves 2 to 4

Calamari nourishes the brain and the blood. It reinforces the spleen and the stomach
and dispels cold.

This dish is often prescribed for women who suffer from amenorrhea, the
abnormal absence or cessation of menses.

2 tablespoons (30 milliliters) cooking oil
2 teaspoons (10 grams) minced ginger
1 pound (500 grams) calamari, cleaned and sliced
1 tablespoon (15 milliliters) cooking wine
1 teaspoon (5 grams) salt

Heat the oil in a wok or frying pan. Drop in the ginger. Stir for a few
seconds. Drop in the calamari. Add the cooking wine and stir for 2 to 3
minutes until cooked. Sprinkle with salt and serve.

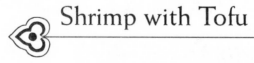

Shrimp with Lettuce

serves 4

Shrimp invigorates the Yang functions and replenishes the essence of the kidneys. Consequently, shrimp is often prescribed as a cure for low sex drive or even impotence. Eating shrimp with lettuce is said to clear skin problems, rendering the skin smooth and elastic. Asthma sufferers are also advised to eat this dish in abundance.

1 pound (500 grams) fresh shrimp, cleaned, peeled, and deveined
1 egg white, beaten
1 tablespoon (15 grams) cornstarch
$^{1}/_{2}$ teaspoon (2.5 grams) salt
$1^{1}/_{2}$ teaspoons (8 grams) minced ginger
2 scallions, minced
12 leaves iceberg lettuce
2 tablespoons (30 milliliters) cookingoil
1 tablespoon (15 milliliters) water
1 teaspoon (5 milliliters) sesame oil

Mince the shrimp and place in a medium-to-large bowl with the egg white, cornstarch, and salt. Mix well.

Mix the ginger and scallions together in a small bowl.

Clean the lettuce leaves and trim to round them off. Arrange the lettuce leaves on a serving plate.

Heat the cooking oil in a wok or frying pan. Throw in the shrimp–egg mixture along with the ginger–scallion mixture. Stir-fry over medium heat for 2 to 3 minutes. Add the tablespoon of water and stir. Stir in the sesame oil and remove from heat. Transfer to a serving plate.

Present the two plates, one of lettuce leaves and one of minced shrimp, separately at the table. Have each diner place a mound of shrimp inside a lettuce leaf and roll it up to eat it from the hand.

Shrimp with Tofu

serves 2 to 3

This dish strengthens Yang, invigorates the functions of the kidneys, and stimulates the appetite. Shrimp is usually prescribed for male sexual problems, such as premature ejaculation and impotence.

4 ounces (125 grams) fresh shrimp, cleaned, peeled, and deveined
1 tablespoon (15 milliliters) cooking wine
Pinch of salt

1 tablespoon (15 grams) cornstarch
2 tablespoons (30 milliliters) plus ¹/₄ cup (60 milliliters) water
1 tablespoon (15 milliliters) cooking oil
8 ounces (250 grams) tofu, cut into 1-inch cubes
1 teaspoon (5 milliliters) sesame oil

In a medium bowl, mix the shrimp with the cooking wine and a pinch of salt. In a small bowl, mix together the cornstarch and the 2 tablespoons (30 milliliters) of water.

Heat the cooking oil in a wok or frying pan. When the oil is hot, add the tofu cubes and stir-fry for 1 minute, then add the ¹/₄ cup (60 milliliters) of water. Lower the heat, cover the wok, and simmer for 5 minutes.

Add the shrimp and stir. Simmer for another 3 minutes. Now add the cornstarch mixture. Stir.

Sprinkle with the sesame oil and stir well. Remove from heat and serve.

Celery Shrimp

serves 2 to 3

This dish replenishes the essence of the kidneys and subdues hyperactivity of the liver. It also brings down swelling, counteracts dizziness and headaches, regulates blood pressure, and alleviates dehydration.

Shrimp are considered a valid remedy for male sexual weaknesses, such as premature ejaculation, over-frequent nocturnal emission, and low sex drive.

1 tablespoon (15 milliliters) cooking oil, or more as needed
5 garlic cloves, peeled and crushed
4 ounces (125 grams) fresh shrimp, cleaned, peeled, and deveined
¹/₂ cup (100 grams) celery, chopped into 1-inch-long pieces
Salt and pepper to taste

Heat the oil in a wok or frying pan. When the oil is hot, add the garlic and stir-fry for 10 seconds, then add the shrimp and stir-fry for 3 minutes. Transfer the shrimp to a bowl and set aside.

Reheat the wok, adding a little more oil or a tablespoon of water if needed. Add the celery segments and stir-fry for 3 minutes.

Return the cooked shrimp to the pan. Stir thoroughly. Add salt and pepper to taste, remove from heat, and serve.

Oysters in Black Bean Sauce

serves 4

Oysters are renowned throughout the world for their aphrodisiac effects. As is often the case with aphrodisiacs, however, these effects exist more in the mind than in the oysters.

Chinese medicine does not emphasize any specific aphrodisiac function in oysters, but it does regard them as a general tonic that may lead to a stronger sex urge. According to Chinese theory, oysters do, in fact, consolidate the vital energy—the qi—of the kidneys, thereby arresting frequent nocturnal seminal emission.

Oysters also nourish the heart, the blood, and Yin essence. They reduce phlegm and soothe the nerves, thus curing such problems as insomnia and nervous sweating.

1 pound (500 grams) oysters, shelled
1 tablespoon (15 grams) cornstarch
2 tablespoons (30 milliliters) plus 4 cups (1 liter) water
2 tablespoons (30 milliliters) cooking oil
2 or 3 garlic cloves, peeled and crushed
1 tablespoon (15 grams) crushed ginger
1 tablespoon (15 grams) black bean sauce
3 scallions, chopped
2½ tablespoons (38 milliliters) soy sauce or oyster sauce
Salt to taste

Wash the oysters under running water and drain them. Examine the oysters for size. They should be small enough to fit easily in the mouth or to be lifted using chopsticks. If they are too large, cut them in half.

In a small bowl, mix the cornstarch with the 2 tablespoons (30 milliliters) of water and set aside.

Fill a medium saucepan with the 4 cups (1 liter) of water, set over high heat, and bring to a boil. When the water is boiling, throw in the oysters. Remove oysters from the water after 20 seconds.

Heat the cooking oil in a wok or frying pan. When the oil is hot, add the crushed garlic, the crushed ginger, and the black bean sauce. Stir-fry for 10 seconds, then add the oysters, scallions, and soy sauce or oyster sauce. Stir for 1 minute, then add the cornstarch mixture and stir well. Add salt to taste. Remove from heat and serve.

Fish with Spinach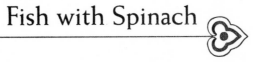

serves 2 to 4

This dish is good for the liver. It also combats high blood pressure, poor appetite, dizziness, and chronic headache.

8 ounces (250 grams) lean fish (cod, snapper, or sole), cut into 1-inch cubes
4 cups (1 liter) water
1 cup (200 grams) packed fresh spinach, in 2-inch-long pieces
2 tablespoons (30 milliliters) cooking oil
3 garlic cloves, peeled and chopped
1 teaspoon (5 grams) chopped ginger
2 scallions, chopped
1 tablespoon (15 milliliters) cooking wine
¹/₂ teaspoon (2.5 grams) salt

In a medium saucepan, bring the water to a boil. Drop the spinach into the boiling water, boil for 30 seconds, then drain and set aside.

Heat the cooking oil in a wok or frying pan over high heat. When the oil is hot, drop in the garlic, ginger, and scallions. Stir for a few seconds and add the fish. Add the cooking wine. Stir for 1 minute and add the spinach. Cover the wok, reduce heat, and simmer for 1 minute.

Add salt and stir well. Remove from heat and serve.

TEAS

Tea, what we call *chia* in China, usually refers to an infusion made with the leaves of the *Camellia sinensis* plant, which is drunk without milk, sugar, or other additives. In China this refreshing drink accompanies meals and, indeed, the activities of most people's entire day.

The following infusions are made from other ingredients in addition to tea leaves. They have specific medicinal properties but, if you like their flavor, they may also be enjoyed simply as beverages. The proportions given in most recipes are for one person. Note that you should always cover the cup or pot when steeping or brewing the tea, lest the volatile oils and other active ingredients escape into the air.

Black Sesame Tea

This tea nourishes the blood, liver, and kidneys and cures bouts of dizziness. It is often prescribed for premature gray hair, pain in the knees, and pain in the lumbar region of the back.

1 teaspoon (5 grams) black sesame seeds
¹/₂ teaspoon (2.5 grams) green tea leaves
1 cup (250 milliliters) water

Heat a dry wok or frying pan and roast the sesame seeds in it for 1 minute. Remove the sesame seeds from the wok. Grind them into a powder using a grinder or a mortar and pestle.

Mix the powder and the tea leaves together.

Bring the water to a boil. Pour the boiling water over the sesame–tea mixture, cover, and brew for 5 minutes.

Ginseng Tea

This tea nourishes the wu zang (the five generating and storing organs of the body—heart, liver, spleen, lungs, and kidneys). Ginseng tea soothes the nerves and stimulates the production of body fluids. It is prescribed specifically for general weakness and exhaustion after childbirth, illness, or surgery, and as a tonic for the elderly.

Caution: You should not drink this tea when you eat daikon or radish, as they weaken the ginseng's effects.

4 fine slices ginseng root
1 cup (250 milliliters) water

Bring the water to a boil. Pour the water over the sliced ginseng, cover, and brew for 10 to 15 minutes.

Drink immediately.

Dry Dandelion and Chrysanthemum Tea

This infusion dissipates toxic heat and evil wind and treats colds as well as sore throats.

3 teaspoons (15 grams) dry dandelion leaves
2 teaspoons (10 grams) dry chrysanthemum flowers
2 teaspoons (10 grams) tea leaves
1 cup (250 milliliters) water

Mix the dandelion leaves, the chrysanthemum flowers, and the tea leaves together. Put 1 heaped teaspoon (5 grams) in a cup.

Bring the water to a boil. Pour the water over the flower–tea mixture, cover, and brew for 5 minutes.

Drink immediately.

Barley Tea

A typical summer drink in China, barley tea has a cooling effect. It is given to people who have suffered from sunstroke and heat exhaustion. It also prevents and cures indigestion.

4 teaspoons (20 grams) barley
1¹/₂ cup (375 milliliters) water

Heat a dry wok or frying pan and roast the barley for 5 minutes, stirring continuously. When done, put the roasted barley in a cup.

Bring the water to a boil. Pour over the roasted barley, cover, and brew for 10 to 15 minutes.

This tea can be drunk either hot or cold.

Ginger Tea

Ginger tea dispels cold, strengthens the functions of the stomach and intestines, and blocks diarrhea. It is also a valid remedy for stomachache.

2 teaspoons (10 grams) minced ginger
2 teaspoons (10 grams) green tea leaves
1¹/₂ cups (375 milliliters) water

Place the ginger, tea leaves, and water in a small saucepan. Bring to a boil, reduce heat to low, cover, and decoct for 10 minutes.
Drink hot.

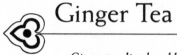# Rose Petal Tea

This tea stimulates qi and blood circulation and soothes the liver. It is a useful remedy for stomachache, breathing difficulties, and menstrual problems.

1 teaspoon (5 grams) dried rose petals, or jasmine petals
1¹/₂ cups (375 milliliters) water

Bring the water to a boil. Pour the boiling water over the dried petals, cover, and brew for 10 minutes.
Drink immediately.

Mint and Chrysanthemum Tea

A good summer drink, this tea dispels heat, soothes the liver, improves eyesight, and aids digestion.

1 teaspoon (5 grams) dry chrysanthemum flowers
2 teaspoons (10 grams) sugar
2 cups (500 milliliters) water
1 teaspoon (5 grams) chopped mint

Place the chrysanthemum and sugar together in a saucepan with the water. Bring to a boil, reduce heat to low, cover, and simmer for 10 minutes.

Add the mint and simmer for another 10 minutes. Drink immediately.

Ginseng and Walnut Tea

This tea nourishes qi, strengthens the functions of the kidneys, and moistens the lungs. It is prescribed for shortness of breath, nervous sweating, dizziness, and tinnitus (ringing in the ears).

4 fine slices ginseng root
3 walnuts, shelled and broken into pieces
4 cups (1 liter) water

Place the ginseng and the walnuts in a saucepan with the water. Bring to a boil over high heat. Lower the heat and simmer for 45 minutes, or until liquid reduces to 1 cup.

Drink immediately.

Fig Tea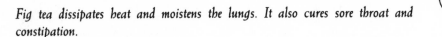

Fig tea dissipates heat and moistens the lungs. It also cures sore throat and constipation.

1 cup (200 grams) fresh figs
2 cups (500 milliliters) water
Sugar, to taste

Wash the figs. Place them in a saucepan with water and bring to a boil. Reduce heat to low, cover the pan, and simmer for 20 minutes.

Strain and drink the juice as a tea. Add sugar as you like.

Mung Bean Tea

A cooling tea that is frequently drunk in China during hot weather, mung bean tea removes heat and dispels thirst and dryness in the throat and mouth. It is used as a remedy in cases of heat exhaustion and sunstroke and is also an effective diuretic. Finally, it lowers blood pressure and is said to improve eyesight.

4 cups (1 liter) water
¹/₂ cup (100 grams) green mung beans
Honey or sugar to taste

In a medium saucepan, bring the water to a boil. Add the mung beans, cover, and boil for 20 to 30 minutes.

Mung bean tea is best drunk cold, but not iced, with a little honey or sugar. The beans are usually eaten too.

WINES

The term "wine," *jiu* in Chinese, refers not to European grape wine but to spirits—generally rice spirits or that of sorghum or other grains.

The wines described below are suitable as after-dinner drinks. Their function is not merely curative; they can be taken for prevention, as a tonic, or simply for the enjoyment of their flavor.

A medicinal dosage for these wines is 2 teaspoons (10 milliliters) two times a day. Wine that is used for medicinal purposes, normally a white wine, should be kept between 50°F and 60°F.

Walnut, Almond, and Jujube Wine

This wine stimulates blood circulation and improves complexion, reinforces qi, and stops premature graying of the hair. It is good for shortness of breath and lower back pain, and for lack of energy due to deficiency of the lungs and the kidneys.

¼ cup (50 grams) almond meats
Water for soaking
½ cup (100 grams) walnut meats
½ cup (100 grams) jujube (Chinese dates)
4 cups (1 liter) rice wine, or sake

Soak the almonds in hot water for 2 hours and remove the skin.

Use a mortar and pestle or stone grinder to grind the almonds and the walnuts into a powder. Put the powder in a large (at least 4-pint or 2-liter) bottle along with the jujube. Add the rice wine, seal the bottle, and let stand to macerate for at least 20 days before drinking.

American Ginseng Wine

This ginseng wine strengthens qi, nourishes Yin, and stimulates the production of body fluids. It is prescribed for weakness, dizziness, shortness of breath, dryness in the mouth and throat, and dry coughs.

¼ cup (50 grams) American ginseng, finely sliced
4 cups (1 liter) rice wine, or sake

Place the ginseng in a bottle with the rice wine.

Seal the bottle and let stand to macerate for at least 15 days before drinking.

Fresh Cherry Wine

Prescribed for weakness, arthritis, and numbness of the legs and arms, this wine strengthens qi, nourishes the blood, dispels wind, and resolves dampness.

2 cups (400 grams) fresh cherries
4 cups (1 liter) rice wine, or sake

Wash the cherries and place them in a bottle with the rice wine.
    Seal the bottle and let the wine stand to macerate for at least 15 days before drinking.

Ginger Wine

Ginger wine strengthens qi, harmonizes the stomach, and arrests nausea and vomiting. It also dispels cold and mitigates wai yin, or external causes of disease. It is beneficial for regulating menstrual periods.

¹/₂ cup (100 grams) ginger, finely minced
¹/₄ cup (60 grams) orange peel, finely minced
¹/₂ cup (100 grams) sugar
4 cups (1 liter) rice wine, or sake

Place the ginger, orange peel, and sugar in a bottle with the rice wine.
    Seal the bottle and let stand to macerate for at least 10 days before drinking.

Rose Petal Wine

This wine stimulates blood circulation and normalizes the flow of qi in the body. Its specific functions are to heal bruises and swellings due to trauma, to regulate menses when there is either too little or too much blood, to relieve a bloated stomach, and to mitigate shortness of breath.

1 cup (200 grams) fresh rose petals
¹/₂ cup (100 grams) sugar
4 cups rice wine, or sake

Place the rose petals in a bottle along with the sugar and rice wine.
    Seal the bottle and let stand to macerate for at least 10 days before drinking.

241

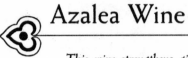

Azalea Wine

This wine strengthens qi, loosens phlegm, and alleviates catarrh. It also treats coughs.

> **¹/₄ cup (50 grams) azalea flowers**
> **4 cups rice wine, or sake**

Wash the azalea flowers and place them in a shaded area to dry. When dry, chop the flowers. Place the chopped flowers inside a bottle with the rice wine.

Seal the bottle and let the wine stand to macerate for 5 days before drinking.

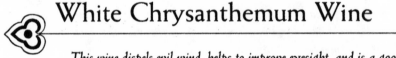

White Chrysanthemum Wine

This wine dispels evil wind, helps to improve eyesight, and is a good treatment for headaches and head colds.

> **¹/₂ cup (100 grams) chrysanthemum flowers**
> **4 cups (1 liter) rice wine, or sake**

Place the flowers in a bottle with the rice wine.

Seal the bottle and let the wine stand to macerate for at least 10 days before drinking.

Dandelion Wine

This is a recipe recorded in Li Shi Zhen's sixteenth century materia medica. This wine dissipates toxic heat and relieves all swellings and skin infections. It stimulates lactation after childbirth. It also cures the intital symptoms of acute mastitis.

¹/₄ cup (50 grams) dandelion leaves
2 cups (500 milliliters) rice wine, or sake

Wash and dry the dandelion leaves. Chop them and place them in a bottle with the rice wine.

Seal the bottle and let the wine stand to macerate for at least 10 days before drinking.

Honeysuckle Vine Wine

This wine dissipates toxic heat and stimulates blood circulation. If taken early it also blocks suppurative infections of the skin.

¹/₂ cup (100 grams) honeysuckle vine
2 tablespoons (30 grams) licorice root
2 cups (500 milliliters) water
1 cup (250 milliliters) rice wine, or sake

Place the honeysuckle vine and licorice in a saucepan with the 2 cups of water. Bring to a boil over medium heat. Continue to boil for about 40 minutes, until only about one-quarter of the water is left. Strain, reserving the liquid, and discard the solid portion.

Pour the reserved liquid from the decoction into a bottle and add the wine.

This wine may be drunk immediately, or at any time after preparation.

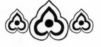

Chapter 7

EXERCISING FOR HEALTH

Everybody in China exercises. School children exercise collectively once a day. Adolescents and young adults go in for wushu and Shaolin boxing. Parents jog, swim, walk, bicycle, and swing weights. Grandparents perform early morning tai ji quan or take a radio to a park for a spot of geriatric disco dancing. Great-grandparents twirl metal spheres in the palms of their hands to exercise their fingers (and the acupuncture points on the hands) or swing their pet canaries' cages as they stroll in the park. But the exercise everybody recognizes as the best for overall fitness and health is one that the Chinese people have been practicing for at least three thousand years. It is qi gong.[1]

Qi corresponds to the Sanskrit word *prana* and the Greek *pneuma;* it means "breath," or "breath of life." The word also refers to material energy, vital matter, the earth's atmosphere, or the fundamental sub-

stance of material beings. The word *gong* translates as "mental control over the body." *Qi gong* thus means "mental control over the flow of qi in one's body. "

Various techniques for exercising control of qi have developed over the centuries. Many of these techniques are medical; others branched out into various disciplines of martial arts. There are Buddhist techniques, Taoist techniques, and Confucian techniques. Fundamentally, however, qi gong may be divided into two basic methods of exercising: *nei dan* and *wai dan,* which respectively mean "internal elixir" and "external elixir."

Nei dan, or internal qi gong, consists of breathing deeply while concentrating on circulating qi inside the body. Wai dan, or external qi gong, is the practice of stimulating certain areas of the body by means of movement and exercise so that qi builds up and flows outward.

Nei Dan Qi Gong

In China it is said that where the mind focuses the qi will follow. Therefore, during nei dan the mind focuses the incoming breath and sends it to the dan tian, the center of all bodily energy, thought to be situated in the lower abdomen. The abdominal muscles are strengthened by the breathing exercises, and more energy is generated. When sufficient qi has accumulated in the dan tian, the mind directs this energy through the two major qi channels, the *ren mei* and *du mei*, which are said to be situated at the front and back of the torso respectively. This practice is referred to as the small circulation of qi, or *xiao zhou tian*. When one is proficient at the small circulation technique, one may then generate stronger qi that is made to flow through all twelve energy channels in the body and limbs in what is known as the *da zhou tian*, or grand circulation. This is said to result in perfect fitness and health.

The first step in the above exercise is to find a good position that allows for correct abdominal breathing. According to some teachers, the best position for practicing internal circulation of qi is sitting with legs crossed. They explain that it is useful to keep the legs crossed because, when you are trying to circulate the qi around the torso (in the small circulation exercise), it can easily go shooting off down your legs unless you obstruct the entrance to the lower channels in the legs by crossing them.

Later, when the grand circulation is attempted, qi is supposed to flow through all the limbs. Therefore, a standing position becomes necessary. This position is the one most frequently used by practitioners of qi gong in China (figure 1).

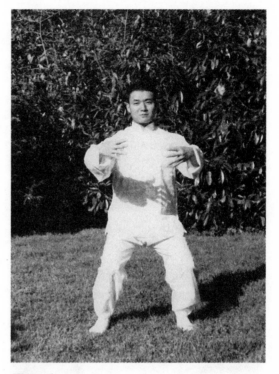

Figure 1

Stand with your feet shoulder-width apart, toes pointing slightly inward. Bend your knees slightly, as if you were about to sit down; the weight of your body should be on your feet and lower legs, not on your thigh muscles. Hold your back and neck straight and raise your arms, bending them at the elbows, as if to encircle a large balloon. Your fingers should be splayed in this same balloon-encircling position. Do not raise your shoulders. Your body should feel relaxed and comfortable.

This position strengthens the muscles of the back, legs, arms, and abdomen. Take care, however, not to overexert yourself in the beginning. The position may look easy but, because of the unusual angle of the legs, a good deal of strain is put on the thighs as well as on the arms. Ten minutes of this position can leave one feeling quite weak. Gradually increase your time spent in the position.

Xiao Zhou Tian (Small Circulation Abdominal Breathing)

There are two techniques for *xiao zhou tian* abdominal breathing—one is Buddhist and the other Taoist. Both employ a cross-legged seated pose (figure 2), although with experience they may also be done standing.

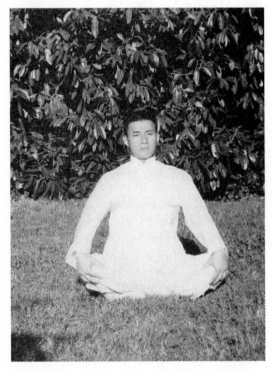

Figure 2

The Buddhist technique consists of focusing on the abdomen while breathing slowly and uniformly through your nostrils. Expand your abdomen as you breathe in; contract it as you breathe out. Do not hold your breath.

The Taoist technique is the opposite of the Buddhist. You concentrate on your abdomen, as above, but you contract it when you inhale and expand it when you exhale. This Taoist breathing technique also goes by the name of *fan hu xi*, or reverse breathing.

Abdominal expansion should never be forced, but should be perfected gradually, with gentle daily practice, until you can expand your abdomen from your navel to your pubic bone.

Once this has been achieved you should sit in quiet meditation, concentrating on your breathing. Imagine the breath traveling through your nose and down to the dan tian, as if you were swallowing something and you could feel it descending all the way to your navel. After a few sittings you should begin to feel a tingling sensation and warmth in the abdominal area. This means that your qi has accumulated sufficiently and that you are now ready to attempt the circulation aspect of the exercise. This is done by guiding the qi around your torso with your mind. At first it will only be a question of imagination and little qi. With time, however, the flow of qi will become stronger and thus more perceptible.

Begin by guiding your qi in the following breathing sequence:

1. Close your mouth and eyes. Press your tongue against your palate. Inhale and guide the incoming qi through your nose and down to the dan tian. Tighten your anal sphincter muscles during the inhalation.
2. Exhale and guide the qi from the dan tian through the groin and into the cavity in front of the coccyx, or tailbone.

This is called the *wei lu* cavity. Relax your anal sphincter as you exhale.

3. Inhale and guide the qi to the base of your neck, between your shoulders.

4. During the final exhalation, guide the qi from the back of your neck to your ears, and then down to your nose and mouth. When the qi enters your mouth, relax your tongue from its position against the roof of your mouth.

One full cycle of xiao zhou tian thus includes two respirations.

You should continue the small circulation exercise for ten minutes two or three times a day. After three months of regular practice you should be ready to go on to the grand circulation exercise.

These exercises are beneficial to the lungs, abdominal viscera, heart, and nervous system.

Da Zhou Tian
(Grand Circulation
Abdominal Breathing)

You are ready to go on to the da zhou tian only when you are confident that you are able to circulate qi around your torso, as in the small circulation exercise. Evidence that you are able to do this correctly consists of a feeling of warmth in all the areas of your body through which your qi is being guided by your mind.

Your pose for the first phase of the grand circulation technique should be either sitting in a chair or standing, preferably in the qi gong standing position. Your thumb and little finger should be touching.

1. Breathe in while contracting your abdomen (or expanding it, if you prefer the Buddhist method of respiration).

Guide the qi from your nose to the dan tian. Tighten the anal sphincter muscles.

2. Exhale and guide the qi to the wei lu in the coccyx. Relax your sphincter muscles.

3. Inhale while guiding the qi to the back of your neck, between the shoulders.

4. During the final exhalation do not guide the qi over the top of your head to your nose as previously, but direct it from the shoulders to your hands and fingers.

Repeat this cycle through several sittings until you feel a warm flow of qi to the center of your palms.

In order to guide the flow of qi to your lower limbs, the usual procedure is followed except that you should adopt a supine position. By lying down and relaxing your leg muscles, the qi is said to flow with greater ease. A standing position will not obstruct the flow of qi completely, but simply constrains the channels a little more.

1. Breathe in as before, guiding the qi from the nose to the dan tian. Exhale and guide the qi through your groin, down your legs, to the center of the soles of your feet.

2. On your subsequent inhalation and exhalation, take the qi up your back and over your head to your nose.

You know that the da zhou tian has been achieved when you are able to feel the warmth of the flowing qi both in your hands and your feet. Your feet may feel hot and numb for several days after you have successfully directed your qi to them. However, do not expect results too quickly. It will take months, at least, to circulate your qi successfully to your hands and feet. Later you will be able to guide the qi to both your hands and feet simultaneously, and direct the qi to any part of your body at will. You will not only be able to cure your own ailments, but you will be able to expand your qi beyond your own body, transmitting it to others and thereby healing their illnesses.

After completing a session of nei dan qi gong, most people need to release some of the energy they have been controlling. This can be done through massage of the limbs, face, and head, or by means of movement exercises such as stretching, turning the head from side to side, or rotating the shoulders.

WAI DAN QI GONG

Most people prefer to train the qi by means of external elixir techniques, or wai dan. Wai dan qi gong does not have to follow nei dan breathing techniques. It may be practiced before them or entirely independently.

Wai dan qi gong techniques involve many complex movements that are not easy to learn from a book. To try to do so would inevitably lead to mistakes in practice. Without a qualified teacher's guidance, a student cannot know if his posture, his sequences, and his speed are correct. Schools of martial arts exist in most towns and cities in America. If you would like to take your study of Oriental breathing techniques further and to practice wai dan qi gong, you should enroll in one of these courses.

However, a short description of one of the earliest forms of wai dan qi gong will do no harm. This practice was taught by the Indian Buddhist monk Bodhidharma, who traveled to China in the sixth century A.D.[2] Bodhidharma was called Da Mo in China, hence the name of this exercise.

When Bodhidharma settled in the Shaolin Buddhist monastery in Henan province in central China in 527 A.D., he is said to have been shocked by the emaci-ated condition of the local monks. As a consequence, he taught them a series of twelve drills based in Indian yoga that ensure fitness and build muscular power as well. These basic drills were later elaborated upon by future generations of monks until they became the world-renowned wushu (literally, "martial" [wu] "art" [shu]) system of Shaolin boxing, also known in English by the Cantonese term kung fu.

The twelve exercises of Da Mo wai dan should be performed in sequence. Each drill consists of at least twenty breaths—energy is built up by relaxing a muscle during inhalation and tensing it during exhalation. By performing the exercises in sequence, the energy built up in one exercise is carried forward to the next. The full sequence of twelve exercises should take about fifteen minutes. Longer sittings would include as many as fifty breaths per drill.

Throughout the Da Mo wai dan exercise you should stand straight with your feet parallel to one another, about twenty-four inches (45 centimeters) apart.

Exercise 1

Stand with your feet approximately two feet apart. Hold your arms by your sides, your elbows slightly bent and your palms open toward the ground (figure 3). Your fingers should be pointing forward. Inhale slowly and uniformly. Exhale and imagine pressing firmly downward with your hands.

In this exercise qi is built up in the wrists.

Exercise 2

Maintain the same position as in exercise 1. Close your hands into fists with your thumbs extended toward your body (figure 4). During exhalation imagine tightening your

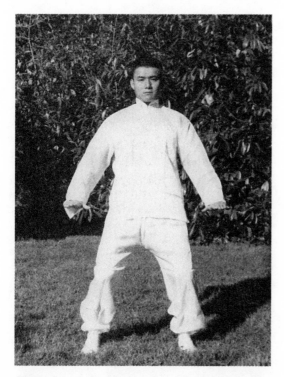

Figure 3

fists and pushing backward with your thumbs. In actual fact, your wrists should only be slightly tensed.

This exercise builds up energy in your hands and fingers.

Exercise 3

Maintain the same position as in exercise 2. Close your thumb over your fingers, making a fist. Turn your fists so the inside of your wrist faces your body (figure 5). Inhale. Then imagine tightening your fists, and exhale.

This exercise builds up energy in the whole of the lower arm.

Exercise 4

Keeping your fists clenched, extend your arms in front of you, the insides of your wrists facing inward (figure 6). Imagine firmly

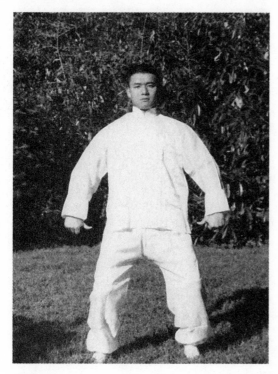

Figure 4

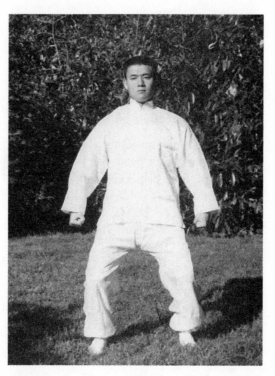

Figure 5

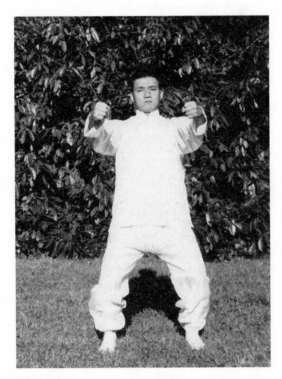

Figure 6

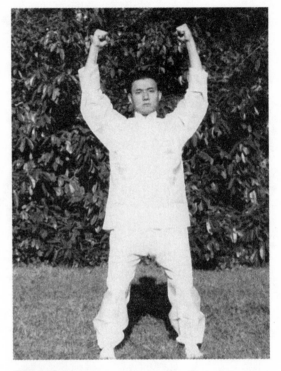

Figure 7

clenching your fists during your exhalation.

This exercise builds qi energy in your chest and shoulders.

Exercise 5

Now raise your arms further until they are straight above your head. Maintain the fist position of your hands (figure 7). Imagine clenching your fists while breathing out.

This exercise builds qi in the shoulders, the neck, and the flanks.

Exercise 6

Bend your elbows and lower your fists to within six inches of your ears. The insides of your wrists should be facing forward (figure 8). Inhale slowly. Exhale and imagine clenching your fists.

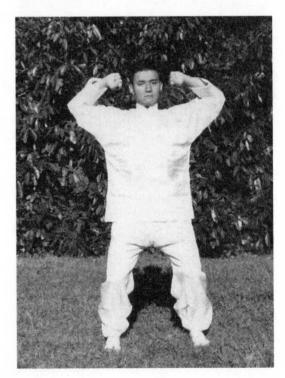

Figure 8

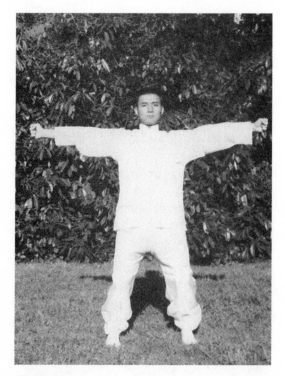

Figure 9

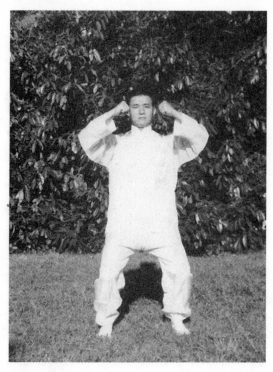

Figure 10

This exercise builds qi in the flanks, the upper torso, and the arms.

Exercise 7

Keeping your fists clenched, extend your arms sideways, parallel to the ground. The insides of your wrists should be facing forward (figure 9). Inhale. Exhale and imagine tightening your fists.

In this exercise, qi builds in the upper torso.

Exercise 8

Bring the extended arms forward. Bend your elbows slightly, giving a circular effect to the position of your arms (figure 10). Imagine clenching your fists during exhalation.

This exercise builds qi in the arms and shoulders.

Exercise 9

Pull your clenched fists back from the previous position, toward your face. Bend your elbows and hold your fists, palms forward, just in front of your cheeks (figure 11). Imagine tightening during your exhalations.

In this exercise, qi is further enhanced in the arms and shoulders.

Exercise 10

Pull your elbows back and raise your forearms so that your fists are held about one foot from either side of your head (figure 12). Imagine clenching your fists during your exhalations.

This exercise is designed to start circulating the qi accumulated in your shoulders.

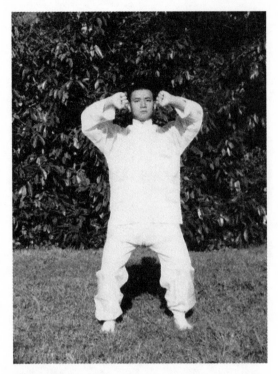

Figure 11

Exercise 11

Keeping your elbows bent as in exercise 10, lower your fists to a position immediately in front of your dan tian, about four inches (10 centimeters) below your navel (figure 13). Imagine clenching your fists during your exhalations, and mentally guide the qi through your arms.

In this exercise qi is no longer accumulated. Instead, the qi already in your body is gathered, and directed to flow through your arms.

Exercise 12

Unclench your fists, straighten your elbows, and raise your arms straight out in front of you. Hold your palms facing skyward (figure 14). When exhaling imagine lifting a heavy weight with your arms.

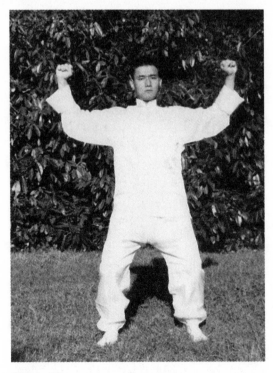

Figure 12

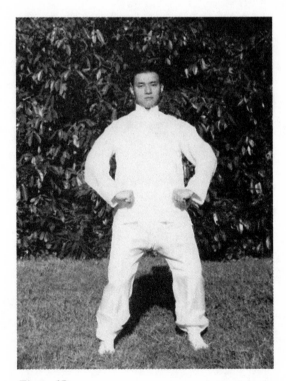

Figure 13

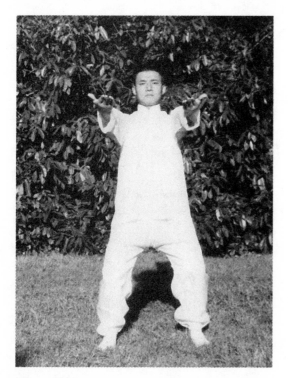

Figure 14

In this exercise, qi is recovered for redistribution around the body.

❖ ❖ ❖

When you have completed the whole wai dan sequence, it is good to relax for a few minutes, either seated or lying down, breathing normally.

Da Mo wai dan qi gong strengthens the body as a whole, and the muscles, joints, and inner organs in particular. These exercises also improve circulation. They ensure the equilibrium of the nervous system, and build up resistance to disease.

There are many other popular wai dan exercises that have derived directly from Bodhidharma's original sequence. One well-known sequence of eight drills, called *ba duan jin*, or Eight Pieces of Brocade, was created by a famous patriotic general, Yue Fei, in the twelfth century, to maintain fit-

ness in the ranks. Yue Fei's ba duan jin was based on an earlier series of exercises by the same name devised by Zhong Li during the Tang dynasty (618–907 A.D.). Other versions of the ba duan jin have been developed over the centuries, some during the last forty years as qi gong started becoming fashionable. Another well-known sequence of qi gong exercises is tai ji quan, an intricate sequence of movements during which the mind guides qi around the body.[3]

Qi gong is becoming ever more popular in the West. Tai ji quan and qi gong lessons are now standard in many health clubs. Together with the increased acceptance of Chinese physical exercise, other aspects of Chinese health systems are also entering Western consciousness. Acupuncture has been used for years in alternative health circles, but is now entering mainstream medical practice. The use of Chinese herbal medicine is becoming increasingly common, to the extent that many allopathic doctors and researchers express interest in discovering the curative properties of these herbs and medicines. Chinese medical theory and practice may still be dismissed by conservatives as mere quackery. Other people extol Chinese traditions beyond all scientific reasonableness, sometimes suggesting curative effects that verge on the miraculous. As is usually the case, the truth lies somewhere between these two extremes.

Chinese traditions spanning millennia cannot be dismissed offhand. Enough empirical and experimental evidence exists to demonstrate that Chinese medical traditions are still valid today. On the other hand, Chinese medicine does not invariably provide a cure whenever Western medicine fails to deliver. What Chinese traditions of healthy living can assure us is that, if we carefully follow their precepts, we can stay healthy and youthful for many years to come.

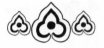

Appendix 1

Daily Requirements of Proteins, Minerals, and Vitamins for the Healthy Adult

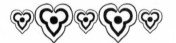

Protein

1 gram of protein for every two pounds of body weight. A person weighing 150 pounds should thus consume 75 grams of protein per day. This amounts to approximately six eggs' worth, or 8 ounces of steak.

Carbohydrates

160–240 grams, equivalent to 300–400 grams of bread (10–14 ounces) or 400–500 grams of rice

Fat

Not more than .25 gram a day for every pound of your ideal body weight, thus if your ideal weight is 150 pounds you should not consume more than 35 grams of fat per

day. Two fried eggs exceed that amount, as do 100 grams (3.5 ounces) of whole-milk cheese. A single cream puff will probably carry a hefty 100 grams of fat.

Fiber

At least 25 grams a day, but the more fiber you eat the better. In the Chinese countryside, 90 grams of fiber a day is considered normal. You would have to eat $1\frac{1}{2}$ pounds of green peas, a high-fiber food, to consume 25 grams of fiber.

Calcium

400–500 milligrams per day, equivalent to one pint of milk. The daily requirement increases to 1000–1400 milligrams during pregnancy and lactation.

Phosphorus

1 gram per day. One hundred grams (3.5 ounces) of meat or mushrooms, or a mere 30 grams (1 ounce) of fish, meets the daily requirement.

Iron

10 milligrams per day. Higher dosages (18 milligrams per day) are necessary for women during their childbearing years (from puberty to menopause), to replenish blood iron lost during menstruation. Iron in the body is used many times over. Intake is necessary only to replenish that which is lost in the feces, during menstruation, or through other blood loss. Women in their childbearing years therefore require more iron than others.

It is dangerous to consume too much iron because excess iron is not easily eliminated. One hundred grams (3$^1/_2$ ounces) of brown bread, meat, spinach, or soybeans contain 2–3 milligrams. One cup of kidney beans contains 5.2 milligrams; 100 grams (3$^1/_2$ ounces) of chives contain 8.5 milligrams; 100 grams of cocoa contains 11.5 milligrams; and 100 grams of pork liver contains 18 milligrams of iron.

Vitamin A

5000 IU (increase to 8000 IU during pregnancy and lactation). Two oranges, one mango, or 10 ounces of cheese would each provide 5000 IU.

Vitamin B₁ (Thiamine)

1.25–1.5 milligrams, equivalent to one bowl of oatmeal or one-half cup of sprouted wheat berries.

Vitamin B₂ (Riboflavin)

1.7–2 milligrams, equivalent to 400 grams (14 ounces) of almonds, or 100 grams (3.5 ounces) of liver.

Niacin

20 milligrams, equivalent to 100 grams (3.5 ounces) of liver, or of peanuts.

Vitamin C (Ascorbic Acid)

60 milligrams, although megadoses (500–1000 milligrams) function as a valid antioxidant. You can get 60 milligrams of vitamin C from a glass of orange juice or a bowl of fresh strawberries; one would have to go about consuming larger quantities more systematically. Remember that vitamin C is destroyed by heat, and decreases with the passage of time between picking and eating.

❖ ❖ ❖

The last five essential vitamins and minerals listed in this table are not included in the nutrient properties of foods discussed in chapter 4. They are nonetheless important to health and wellness, and are therefore included here.

Magnesium

400 milligrams. Magnesium activates an enzyme that allows the absorption of carbohydrates in the body. It is common in greenleaf vegetables and in beans. One-half cup of raw parsley contains 13 milligrams of magnesium, one cup of raw spinach contains 22 milligrams, and 100 grams (3.5 ounces) of stir-fried soybean sprouts contain 28 milligrams.

Iodine

150 micrograms. Iodine is indispensable for the thyroid gland's synthesis of the hormone thyroxine. It is found in soil and most underground water supplies and is absorbed into the body by consuming vegetables grown in an iodine-rich soil. In areas lacking iodine in the soil, goitre, a swelling of the neck due to iodine deficiency, used to be common. Nowadays most brands of table salt have added iodine. Iodine deficiency is therefore extremely rare.

Copper

2 milligrams. Copper appears to aid the action of iron in the formation of red blood corpuscles. Bodily requirements are so low that there is rarely any real danger of deficiency. A two-cup portion of boiled soybeans provides 2 milligrams of copper. Small amounts are found in most foods.

Zinc

15 milligrams.[1] Zinc is essential to the red blood corpuscles for the metabolism of carbon dioxide. It is also an important factor in regulating enzyme production, protein synthesis, muscular contraction, the formation of insulin, and the acid-alkaline balance in the blood. Zinc is found in meat, brewer's yeast, wheat germ, sunflower seeds, and eggs.

Vitamin E

30 IU. Vitamin E is an important antioxidant, indispensable for maintaining cellular efficiency and youthfulness. Wheat germ is the richest source of vitamin E; a single tablespoon provides 20.3 milligrams. Almonds, sweet potatoes, and greenleaf vegetables are also rich in vitamin E.

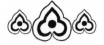

Appendix 2

MAIL-ORDER RESOURCES

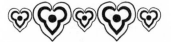

SOURCES OF HERBAL SUPPLIES

The following are mail order suppliers of Chinese herbs and other ingredients. Some of them have minimum orders of $10 to $20.

California

East Earth Trade Winds
P.O. Box 493151
Redding, CA 96049
(800) 258-6878

Great China Herb Company
857 Washington Street
San Francisco, CA 94108
(415) 982-2195
FAX (415) 982-5138

Moonrise Herbs
826 G Street
Arcata, CA 95521
(707) 822-5296

Superior Trading Company
837 Washington Street
San Fransico, CA 94108
(415) 982-8722

Trans Trading Company
849 Washington Street
San Francisco, CA 94108
(415) 788-0110

New York

Chinese Herbal Center
28 Bowery
New York, NY 10013-5100
(212) 732-4548

Lay Hang
220 Centre Street
New York, NY 10013-3632
(212) 431-5636

Lee Bok Kyong
124 W 30th Street
New York, NY 10001-4009
(212) 244-0030

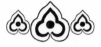

Notes

Introduction

1. In case there are no Oriental markets in your area, addresses of select shops that accept mail orders are included in appendix 2.

2. The one exception is raw bitter apricot kernel, used in a cure for asthma. It is toxic only when eaten raw, and must not be consumed in large quantities or over a long period of time. For more information on bitter apricot kernel, see pages 38 and 69.

3. Some famous medics went as far as to systematically test the effects of all known medical substances on themselves. One of these, Li Shi Zhen (1518–1593), tested 1,892 ingredients and, on the basis of these, went on to prescribe over ten thousand preparations. The result was China's definitive illustrated pharmacopoeia of medicinal ingredients, Li Shi Zen's *Ben Cao Gang Mu* (Compendium of Materia Medica), published in 1590.

4. Many hospitals and clinics in China provide a combination of therapies. Western allopathic cures are prescribed where these work best, and traditional medicines are suggested for chronic conditions that need time and patience to remedy.

Chapter 1

1. The Yellow Emperor was so called not because of the color of his skin but because he ruled over the earth. In Chinese tradition, yellow is the color associated with the Earth element.

2. Oracles written on bovine hip bones and tortoise shells indicate that it was understood as early as the Shang dynasty (c. 1750–1100 B.C.) that disease could arise independently within various organs of the body, or as a result of external causes, such as in the case of an epidemic.

3. Lao tzu is reputed to be the author of the Taoist classic, the *Tao Te Ching* (The Way and Its Power). Zhuang Zi (perhaps recognized more readily by Western readers as Chuang-tzu) was the author of a work bearing his own name that had considerable influence on Chinese Buddhism, landscape painting, and poetry.

4. As is common in English-language writings on traditional Chinese medical theory, the names of the individual Elements are capitalized to remind the reader of the more expansive meanings of the words.

5. The *Lei Jing*, or Systematic Compilation of the Internal Classic, was compiled by Zhang Jie Bin during the late Ming dynasty, in 1624. It is recognized as the most important book of reference in the study of the *Huangdi Nei Jing*.

Chapter 2

1. Although these various causes of illness have been referred to since antiquity, it was not until the Southern Song dynasty (1127–1279) that the three categories of pathology were formally classified. In 1174, Chen Yan (also known as Chen Wu Ze) published an eighteen-volume text, the title of which translates as A Treatise on the Three Categories of Pathogenic Factors of Diseases. He based his classifications on those originally suggested by Zhang Zhong Jing between A.D. 159 and 219 in another of China's most famous medical classics, Synopsis of Prescriptions of the Golden Chamber. Zhang Zhong Jing's three categories of *causa morbi* were:
    1. Endogenous cause of disease, when pathogenic factors invade the channels and collaterals;
    2. Exogenous causes, when external

pathogenic factors invade the four extremities and the nine body orifices and then circulate through the blood vessels, thus obstructing the flow of qi;
    3. Intemperance in sexual life, various traumata, animal and insect bites (from Synopsis of the Golden Chamber, chapter 1, clauses 1–2).

2. Xie qi is often called the *liu yín* or "six aberrations." This *yín* is not the same as the *yin* for cause (as in *wai* and *nei yin*) nor, indeed, as the *yin* of Yin and Yang. It is sometimes translated as "devil."

3. Yin qiao pills are febrifugal pills of lonicera (honeysuckle), forsythia, balloonflower root, burdock fruit, *Lophaterum*, *Schizonepta*, soybean, peppermint, and licorice.

4. The first official pharmacopoeia, which included reference to fungi, was published during the Tang Dynasty in A.D. 659.

5. The first reliable reference to inoculation is by Chen Zhong Yang, who lived during the tenth century A.D. Some authors affirm that the practice actually began in the sixth century.

6. The method was not, of course, without its dangers. Since Pasteur's nineteenth-century discoveries that a virus can be weakened for use as an inoculation, modern Western methods of immunization have entirely taken over in China.

Chapter 3

1. This is true everywhere but in Guangdong (Canton) province in the south, where soup is eaten first, as in Europe and America.

2. The famous dish Cantonese fried rice originated as a way to use leftovers.

When in a hurry, you throw some rice into a pan together with whatever remains from a previous meal.

3. Contrary to popular belief, rice is not the staple dish all over China. It is consumed in larger quantities in the south, where it grows faster. Northern Chinese cuisine tends to prefer wheat (bread or noodles).

4. On average, Chinese people obtain 87 percent of their total calories from plant sources and only 13 percent from animals. In the United States, 39 percent of all calories consumed are obtained from animal sources; in the United Kingdom, foods from animal sources account for 35 percent of all calories consumed. Source: The United Nations Food and Agriculture Organization yearbook. Rome, 1992.

5. A *kang* is the traditional hollow brick platform found in peasant homes. It is heated from the inside. The entire family eats, works, and sleeps on top of the kang during the cold season.

6. This questionnaire is based on one drawn up by Dr. Henry C. Lu in his excellent book *Chinese System of Food Cures: Prevention and Remedies* (New York: Sterling, 1986).

Chapter 4

1. Combining traditional therapies with modern Western medicine is a practice frowned upon by most traditional doctors. Nevertheless, today few people are in fact patient enough to wait for traditional remedies to take full effect. It is common, therefore, particularly among city dwellers, to resort to a quick antibiotic "fix," combining that with traditional food therapies to counteract

resulting toxic imbalances.

2. Tannins and alkaloids react biochemically with protein-based tonics. Although ancient Chinese doctors had no understanding of biochemistry, experience taught them the negative effects of some ingedients when combined with others.

3. Our sources are various nutrition handbooks, including Bowes and Church's *Food Values of Portions Commonly Used,* 15th ed. (New York: Harper and Row, 1989).

4. Ying Jianghe, et. al., *Icones of Medicinal Fungi from China* (Beijing: Science Press, 1987). This book describes 272 varieties of medicinal fungi.

5. Private communication with the president of Italy's rice growers' association. Shortly after our conversation in 1985, this man died of cancer of the liver, caused (it is suspected) by eating too much (poisoned) rice.

6. K. Napier in "Taking Soy to Heart," Harvard Health Letter, November 21, 1995, 1–2.

7. In India beef is not eaten for two basic reasons, both of them economic. First there is the question of space. Cattle need space. Five hundred percent more land is needed to provide the same amount of nutrients from beef as from agriculture. Clearly, therfore, in an overcrowded land like India or China, cattle ranches are not the norm. Second, cattle are more useful to the Indian (and Chinese) peasant alive rather than dead. Cattle pull the plow, provide milk to babies, and turn pumps and grinders, and their dried droppings are used both as insulation and as a smokeless fuel for cooking.

8. As far back as B.C. 4000, a daily ration of garlic was handed out to the workers on

the Great Pyramid of Cheops in Egypt in order to keep them fit and healthy. Garlic was used extensively by the Romans and the ancient Indians. Hippocrates, from the Greek island of Kos, founder of medical science, recommended garlic against infectious disease and for intestinal disorders. Louis Pasteur confirmed its antibiotic effects in 1858.

Finally, a poem written in England in 1607 by Sir John Harrington makes for educational and amusing reading:

Sith garlicke then hath power to save
  from death,
Bear with it though it make unsavoury
  breath.
And scorn not garlicke like some that
  thinke
It only makes men winke and drinke and
  stinke.

9. Drinking an extract of garlic in water appears to slow the growth of bladder cancer in laboratory mice. Dale R. Riggs, Jean I. DeHaven, and Donald J. Lamm, "Allium Sativum (Garlic) Treatment for Transitional Cell Carcinoma," *Cancer* 79, no. 10 (1997): 3.

10. The greatest production of ginseng in the world is in the Kamloops area in southern British Columbia, Canada.

11. The precise date of the first use of tea is not known. We do know, however, that by the first millennium B.C. tea was already an old and well-established drink.

12. According to one story, tea was created by the compassionate Buddha for the benefit of Buddhist monks who fell asleep during meditation. Bodidharma was an Indian monk who went to China in the sixth century A.D. to teach meditation. During an early morning meditation he fell asleep. So angry was he on awakening that he cut off his eyelids. (Bodidharma is always depicted with wide, staring eyes.) The Buddha took pity on him. Where Bodidharma's eyelids had fallen there grew two green plants. The leaves of these plants brewed in hot water would, from that time forward, ensure that Bodidharma and other monks would never again fall asleep during meditation.

13. Chen Junshi, et. al., *Diet, Lifestyle and Mortality in China: A Study of the Characteristics of 5 Chinese Counties*, Beijing: Oxford University Press, Cornell University Press, and People's Medical Publishing House, 1991.

14. Soybeans are low fat, fiber-filled, and able to clear cholesterol from circulation. According to the Harvard Health Letter, regularly eating five ounces of firm tofu may lower bad cholesterol by up to 25 percent. *Medizin* November/December 1996 issue.

15. At the Research Institute of Epidemic Diseases at the Chinese Academy of Science in Beijing.

Chapter 5

1. It is worth pointing out that, although aluminum does enter the bloodstream at what might be considered dangerous levels through cooking in aluminum vessels, a far greater quantity of the metal is ingested every time one swallows a buffered medication—approximately one hundred times as much as is introduced through cooking with aluminum pots.

2. Some of these ancient pots are on display at the Banpo Neolithic archaeological site and museum on the outskirts of Xian.

3. If, when you need to make a decoction, you find that your pot is broken or missing, the customary thing to do is to borrow your neighbor's. You use it until you are cured. When you have finished with it you do not return it; if you were to do so, superstition decrees that you would be passing your ailment on to your neighbor. Instead, when he needs it, and only when he needs it, the neighbor will come to your place to ask for the pot.

4. *Sake* is the Japanese word for rice wine. The Chinese word is *jiu.*

5. *Diet, Lifestyle and Mortality in China.* The figures are: 0.073 to 0.247 mg/dl in Chinese males and 0.064 to 0.146 in Chinese females compared to 0.060 to 0.150 mg/dl and 0.050 to 0.130 in American men and women, respectively. The difference between iron counts in men and women is due to women's blood loss during menstruation.

6. In June, 1997, one of the authors photographed a tiger paw for sale in Guangzhou's (Canton) crowded public market. It was not on display in one of the stalls, but was instead placed on the ground at the end of the market by two men who said that they had traveled to Canton from Xinjiang region, in the remote west of the country. Nobody around them seemed to be disturbed by the nature of their wares.

7. In the West it is widely believed that dogs are eaten in China. However, in actual fact the consumption of dog meat in China is not, by any means, a common occurrence; neither of the authors has ever tasted it or seen it cooked. Only two people of our acquaintance in China have ever eaten dog. One of those people ate it once in his sixty-year-long life because he was suffering from a cold-disease syndrome and because, as he told us, he was curious. The other had eaten dog on half a dozen occasions and boasted that he liked it.

8. Yogurt was first introduced in northern China in the late 1980s. The Chinese took to it at once. Today it is sold at street stalls in all large northern cities. In the south of China (south of the Yangtze River) yogurt is still virtually unknown. A recent response there to my request for yogurt (called *suan nai* [sour milk]) was met with open-mouthed incredulity. "What do you want sour milk for?" I was asked. "It's bad for you!"

9. Milk contains large quantities of the amino acid tryptophan, which is a natural sleep inducer. Other foods containing tryptophan, and which might thus be useful taken before bedtime, are chicken, turkey, tuna fish, beef, cheese, yogurt, and buttermilk.

Traditional Chinese dietary measures for counteracting insomnia do not include milk and dairy products simply because these are not common in China. However, we did hear that a cup of steaming milk is a common nightcap in the central Asian and predominantly Muslim western province of Xin Jiang where milk is an integral part of people's diets.

Chapter 6

1. This is true everywhere but in Guangdong (Canton) province in the south where soups are taken at the start of the meal as in Europe and the United States.

2. World Health Organization Yearbook, Rome, 1989 and 1996.

3. The recent improvements in living standards means that "special occasions" for many families are becoming the norm,

thus leading to an increase in meat eating. This fact is beginning to cause some health concerns among Chinese dietitians and doctors.

Chapter 7

1. The earliest known reference to qi gong is from the Warring States Period (476–221 B.C.) However, there exists pictorial evidence from the Shang and Zhou dynasties (1122–770 B.C.) that qi gong breathing exercises were being used then for medical purposes.

2. Bodhidharma is the founder of the Chan school of Chinese Buddhism. The word *chan* comes from the Sanskrit *dhyan*, which means meditation. *Chan* in Japanese is pronounced **zen**. Bodhidharma can thus be considered the founder of Zen Buddhism.

3. More commonly known in English as tai chi. *Tai ji quan* literally translates as: "the grand ultimate equilibrium," in reference to the Taoist theory of Yin and Yang. The word *quan* means "boxing style."

Appendix 1

1. It was only in 1963 that it was realized that zinc was important to the human metabolism; it took another ten years for RDA guidelines to be issued. Because of the uncertainty regarding zinc, some authorities suggest that 15 milligrams may be too high.

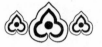

INDEX

THE HEALING CUISINE

India's Art of Ayurvedic Cooking

Harish Johari

The Chinese art of healing with food is matched only by India's equally ancient science of Ayurveda, which views the human being as intimately connected with the environment and all other life forms. Much like China's healing tradition, Ayurveda places great emphasis on diet and the attributes of specific foods. In *The Healing Cuisine*, Harish Johari explains the healing qualities of foods and spices and indicates which combinations are appropriate for various conditions of body and mind. Ten years in the making, this beautiful book is filled with recipes that bring the depth of Ayurvedic knowledge to the delightful experience of preparing and sharing sumptuous meals that feed both body and soul.

ISBN 0-89281-382-2   **$16.95 pb**